Physician Burnout: An Emotionally Malignant Disease

Physician Burnout: An Emotionally Malignant Disease

...

Naim El-Aswad, MD
Zeina Ghossoub, PhD
Relly Nadler, PsyD

ISBN: 1548404632
ISBN 13: 9781548404635
Library of Congress Control Number: 2017910188
CreateSpace Independent Publishing Platform
North Charleston, South Carolina

Preface

. . .

THE PRACTICE OF MEDICINE HAS long been viewed by society as both an art and a science. Not only must practitioners have the knowledge and understanding of diseases and cures, but it is equally important, if not more so, that they master the art of diagnosing, treating, and comforting patients. Those who work in the medical field know that the physician–patient relationship has been, is, and will always be the foundation on which this entire noble profession is based.

It follows that this foundation relies on the interaction of human beings on a physical, emotional, moral, and sometimes spiritual level. The relationship is dynamic, ever evolving, unique, and sacred. But as varied as it is with regard to practitioners, patients, and specialties, the profession is still governed by a defined set of ethical rules and regulations, is dependent on a core group of competencies, and is shaped by economics, politics, government, and judicial law. There is perhaps no other relationship between two individuals that is as scrutinized, closely monitored and controlled, and narrowly steered as the physician–patient relationship.

In recent years, an occult malignancy plaguing the medical community has come to light: physician burnout. Alarmingly, every physician (and other medical professional) is at risk for burnout, and the consequences can be catastrophic. The added challenge with the physician–patient relationship is that not only are physicians severely affected, but the impact of their burnout is felt across patients, families (both of the patient and of the physician), institutions, and the entire human race.

The purpose of this book is to create awareness of physician burnout. Using research and findings, we aim to consolidate the information into a practical, usable format that will provide the medical community and its governing boards with insight and approaches to managing burnout, as well as potential treatments. With all diseases, treatments and cures generally lag until a full understanding of the pathophysiology is achieved. Burnout is no different. Awareness of its prevalence and impact is now being raised nationally and internationally, but what is still missing is a pathway that includes both understanding of the problem and an outline for treatment.

We propose two treatment modalities that have proved scientifically valid and, more importantly, effective across several disciplines and professions, including medicine. These approaches, emotional intelligence (EI) and wellness, will be discussed in the context of burnout and its effects, and how, in the science of EI and the applications of wellness, there is a better understanding of the pathophysiology and treatment of burnout.

Burnout is an indolent malignant existence, and in our study of it, we have identified six concepts that we will explore throughout this book:

1. Burnout as a malignancy
2. The pendulum of burnout
3. Emotional intelligence
4. Optics and burnout
5. Wellness and burnout
6. Balance and burnout

By discussing burnout and actions necessary to manage it, we intend to increase awareness, enhance acknowledgement and acceptance, and offer guidelines and personal-use tools for action on an individual and institutional level.

Chapters

CHAPTER 1

The Physiology of a Physician

• • •

"Wherever the love of medicine is found, there is also love of humanity"

HIPPOCRATES

IN THE MEDICAL FIELD, THE treatment of a disease starts with understanding its pathophysiology, identifying its risk factors, outlining its symptomatic manifestations, creating diagnostic approaches to "read" its signs, and developing both a preventive and a treatment approach. This book is predicated on the philosophy of this approach. As we take you through the journey of burnout, allow us to help you identify it, recognize it, understand it and manage it.

This journey starts with an imaginary scenario. Let us imagine there is a screening test that can detect cancer X and stage it. Now let's suppose that we run this test on every human being in community Y. We discover that 50 percent, or one out of every two people, has cancer X, which has dire effects on health and can be fatal. Now, to make things more dramatic, let's suppose that all of the people afflicted with cancer X are at the advanced terminal stages IIIb or IV.

So, half of all people in community Y have advanced-stage cancer X (stage IIIb or IV).

What do we do?

Now, imagine that this scenario is true. Actually, we do not need to imagine it—because it *is* true! Let's remove the hypothetical names and replace them with real ones. "Cancer X" becomes "burnout," and "Community Y" becomes "the medical community." The real formula then becomes:

Half of all physicians have advanced-stage burnout.

Now, what do we do?

First, we must comprehend how and why burnout is happening, and to do that, we need to start with the affected individual: the physician.

THE PHYSIOLOGY (VIRTUES) OF A PHYSICIAN

"Observation, Reason, Human Understanding,
Courage; these make the physician."

—MARTIN H. FISCHER (1879–1962)

The four virtues listed above are the foundation of the entire physician training system. They are divided and taught along six different competencies as defined by the Accreditation Council for Graduate Medical Education (ACGME) [1]. These competencies are:

1. Professionalism
2. Interpersonal and communication skills
3. Medical knowledge
4. Practice-based learning and development
5. Patient care
6. System-based practice

With evaluation forms and guidelines[1], the ACGME and other medical governing bodies strive to ensure that physicians maintain these competencies throughout their career. There are ethical and clinical guidelines

---

1 Holmboe E.S., Edgar L., Hamstra S. *The Milestones Guidebook.* ACGME publication. 2016.

on how to maintain knowledge and best practice the profession, as well as the requirement of *preserving* the ability to practice the profession to our fullest potential. What is missing from these guidelines are the necessary steps that are needed to help us shield ourselves from the erosion of our cognitive abilities and focus, the loss of meticulousness of our skills, and the breakdown of empathy and compassion that drive us.

No matter a physician's specialty, at the point of interaction with the patient, the four virtues given above are what matter most. Now let's look at them in the context of the three major factors that this book, the medical practice, burnout, and its treatment are based:

1. You as the physician (or medical provider)
2. Your interaction with the patient
3. The patient

From this point forward, we will refer to them as PIP formula (Physician, Interaction, Patient). Further, we will also use the phrase "mastering the moment," which will refer to being fully aware of ourselves and others *at the moment* when we interact with the patient (or the nurse, the staff, other physicians, or the patient's family). In other words, how are we in our emotional and physical state at that time, and are we able to see and understand the patient so we can appropriately manage their care? Mastering the moment is what would ensure the success of the PIP.

Now, look in depth at the above mentioned four virtues of a physician.

OBSERVATION

"The whole art of medicine is in observation..."
"Learn to see, learn to hear, learn to feel, learn to smell,
and know that by practice alone can you become expert.

—WILLIAM OSLER

Everything we do as physicians depends on our abilities of observation and perception. We must be able to not only observe, but also comprehend what we are observing. In medical school, we are trained to use the five senses to do this. Fruity breath, a cool extremity, a trembling hand, and sonorous breaths are all clues, but they can only be understood through the optics of medicine. Observation is a skill in and of itself—a power that is introduced and honed in medical school and then further refined during residency and specialty training. It is put to the test every time a PIP occurs.

However—and this is a big however—what is missing in our training are the tools we need (or the optics we should develop) to evaluate our skills in observation, to ensure we are always performing to the best of our abilities and to maximize the knowledge of our teachings and the expertise of our training. However, the nature of our profession and PIP leads to a decrease in the ability and skills needed for observation, which in turn results in a less than optimal (or even downright dangerous) PIP. With physician burnout, we cannot master the moment, and this ultimately leads to suboptimal, and sometimes dire, outcomes.

So, what does observation rely on? It requires clarity of mind, focus, detailed perception, and an awareness of ourselves and others, as well as relentless, almost obsessive, attention. Observation provides information and insight, and helps us formulate a plan of approach for our PIP, so anything that detracts from the above-mentioned abilities decreases our capability to observe. Since observation is the first element in connecting with patients, taking a history, doing a physical exam, diagnosing an ailment, communicating in an understandable manner, and developing a plan of action, it is crucial that we maintain this capability.

The formula for observation is:

$$O = Cl * F * P * A * K$$

Observation (O) = Clarity (Cl) * Focus (F) *
Perception (P) * Awareness (A) * Knowledge(K)

Some negative effects on observation are: stress (emotional, physical, mental, psychosocial, economical), emotional lability and irritability, cognitive impairment, physical pain and problems, preoccupation with personal problems, and external pressures, to name just a few. With these in mind, take a moment to consider how they relate to your practice and your profession currently. On a scale of 0-10, (least to best), where would you rate yourself? Plug in your own numbers and determine how much of your power of observation, if any, is decreased because of your profession and practice. We have used multiplication here instead of addition because these factors are dependent on each other. They are complimentary and mutually affect each other. When one decreases, all the others are affected. When you evaluate your selves, use these as a way of gaging yourselves on good days and bad days. They are used only as a guideline. Repeat these steps for the remaining formulas discussed below.

REASON
Our cognitive abilities are represented by reason, and we know this because as physicians we are trained in neuroscience and psychiatry. We also learn about the power of reasoning, which relies on the full abilities of our cognitive function. A common theme arises: The entire premise of practicing medicine stands on the maximum output from our six competencies and four virtues.

What factors, then, affect the power of reason? Clarity and focus are two obvious ones, and knowledge and critical thinking would be two more. Physicians are taught, through reason, how to interpret the data they acquire, and how to use medical algorithms that are scientifically valid.

The formula for reason is:

$$\text{Reason (R)} = \text{Clarity (Cl)} * \text{Focus (F)} *$$
$$\text{Knowledge (K)} * \text{Critical Thinking (Cr)}$$
$$R = Cl*F*K*Cr$$

Reason is affected when any of the factors are altered, and when reason is negatively affected, medical practice is not at its optimum.

HUMAN UNDERSTANDING

In a word, human understanding can be described as empathy. It is the ability to see with the eyes of your patient, listen through the ears of your patient and feel with your patient's heart. As physicians and medical providers, we often have people share with us their joys and sorrows. We are there to comfort them, show understanding, and make sure they are cared for both medically and emotionally.

Empathy is a great measure of our humanity and is one of the pillars on which the foundation of medicine is established, but it is also one of the first pillars to crumble when a physician experiences burnout. We will discuss the impact of burnout on empathy in chapter 2, but before we do that, let's review the factors that affect empathy.

Human understanding relies on our humanity—on our emotional well-being and ability to communicate with the patient. We must be able to observe, with all our senses, what the patient is experiencing. At the point of contact (or the moment of communication), it is critical that we communicate the acknowledgement and awareness of what the patient is feeling. In fact, empathy is so important that evaluation systems and feedbacks, payment modalities, and reimbursement (for example, Press Ganey surveys) depend on it. Indeed, a skilled physician who has no empathy will suffer in reputation, in standing, in income, and in value.

The formula for human understanding is:

$$\text{Human Understanding (HU)} = \text{Humanity (H)} *$$
$$\text{Emotional Well-being (EW)} * \text{Communication (Co)}$$
$$HU = H*EW*Co$$

Now, take a moment and look at these factors within yourself. Analyze your good days and your bad days, then make a list of what affects your HU.

COURAGE

The last virtue is courage. In medicine, we define it as the ability to express ourselves freely, to practice accurately and professionally, to withstand the weight of dealing with human lives and health, and to accept our own limitations and vulnerabilities. Courage outcome can be measured through the medical data of morbidity and mortality and how we react to them, but at its core, it is the final translation of our profession.

Our training aims to make us comfortable with our decisions. The practice of medicine is not for the faint of heart, nor should it be taken lightly. There is a fine line between courage and arrogance, between humility and hubris. Maintaining that balance, and staying on the positive side of courage, is what the practice of medicine is all about.

The factors affecting courage are knowledge and skills, professionalism and emotional expression, ethical and moral awareness, and a deep, realistic understanding of our abilities and limitations. Courage depends on us being truthful with ourselves and honest with our conclusions.

The formula for courage is:

$$\text{Courage (Cu)} = \text{Knowledge (K)} * \text{Professionalism (P)} *$$
$$\text{Emotional Expression (E)} * \text{Moral awareness (M)}$$
$$Cu = K*P*E*M$$

Now, take a big step back and assess the courage of yourself and your medical practice.

BURNOUT AND THE PHYSICIAN

No matter what formula you use or believe in, no matter what factors you believe affect the PIP, there are some universal truths that will be stressed throughout this book:

1. The practice of medicine is dependent on emotional and cognitive abilities.

2. Burnout can affect any and all of the six ACGME competencies and the four virtues of a physician.
3. The effect of burnout comes through the factors listed in the above formulas.
4. Any intervention must account for and target these same factors.

Burnout and the factors leading to it will ultimately impact our ability to master the moment of interaction with the patient. Therefore, anything and everything we can do to minimize the effect of burnout and protect against it is translated into decreased morbidity and mortality, both for physicians and their patients.

CHAPTER 2

The Pathophysiology of Burnout

• • •

"Burnout is what happens when you try
avoiding being human for too long."

— MICHAEL GUNGOR

WHILE WORKING IN THE EMERGENCY room in 2009, I met a new graduate (we will call him Dr. Smith) who had just finished his residency and was starting as an attending. Our work stations were next to each other, and I often overheard him patiently explain to a nurse the pathophysiology of a certain disease, or watched him take the time to talk in depth with a patient. Dr. Smith was a warm, delightful man to work with, and all the staff loved him and raved about his bedside manner, demeanor, composure, and clinical judgment. He was a "solid" physician.

Fast-forward to 2014 and, after several years of not working with Dr. Smith, our paths crossed again. During this shift, I worked with a very different Dr. Smith. He yelled at the nurses, cursed out the staff, and called his patients unflattering names. He was judgmental, downright angry with patients just for showing up, and when someone questioned him about a clinical decision, he became defensive, rude, and aggressive.

Sadly, this transformation of a physician is not at all uncommon in the medical profession. In this book, we will walk you through the issues that led Dr. Smith, version 2009, to become Dr. Smith, version 2014 (the "pathophysiology" part of the book). We will then expound on the rationale and method for returning a physician (or other healthcare professional) to optimum performance (the "treatment" part of the book).

A Slow and Silent Cancer

10-20 years ago, discussing burnout would have been taboo. It is still considered a taboo till this day in the medical world. Further, finding a credible reference on the topic would have been nearly impossible. But in recent years there has been a sudden explosion of interest in burnout, in all parts of the medical field and across all healthcare professionals. The extreme consequences of burnout are now so obvious that the general public and the medical society have no choice but to acknowledge its signs, symptoms, prevalence, and, perhaps most important of all, potential treatment. It has also become increasingly evident that physicians—those who are often diagnosing the burnout in the public—are not protected against it, nor do they have the ability to recognize it in themselves or the tools to combat it and prevent it.

In the simplest of analogies, burnout can be likened to a cancer that slowly and silently grows within us; by the time it is noticed, it may be too late or too advanced to treat. According to Dr. James Suliburk, an associate professor of surgery at the Baylor College of Medicine in Houston, Texas, "burnout creeps on you." He also points out a dangerous aspect of this burnout malignancy: it is contagious! Now there is an urgent push, bordering on critical, to identify burnout's risk factors, stage it, analyze it, and develop a treatment for it.

According to Tait D. Shanafelt M.D. et al. in 2015, burnout is characterized by exhaustion of emotions, a sense of lack of meaning in work, feeling ineffective, and a propensity to view patients and people as objects rather than human beings.[2] What should be stressed are the relationship

---

2 Shanafelt T.D., Hasan O., Dyrbye L.N., Sinsky C., Satele D., Sloan J., West CP. (2015) Changes in Burnout and Satisfaction With Work-Life Balance in Physicians and the General US Working Population Between 2011 and 2014. *Mayo Clinic Proceedings.* 90(12), 1600-13.

to and roots of burnout in the emotional state and well-being. Such a relationship will be further clarified as we discuss the tools needed for diagnosing, preventing, and treating burnout.

Burnout develops over time. Its chronic nature makes it difficult to detect until acute features manifest, such as explosion of emotions, erratic behavior, suicidal thoughts, alcohol abuse, or compassion fatigue. And since burnout is an emotional disease, any aspect of it that is linked to the medical profession and has the potential to negatively affect us emotionally is a risk factor. Universally, factors affecting our emotions illicit a reaction we refer to as "stress." For physicians, stress factors can result from many issues, including:

1. Potential harm to the patient
2. Inability to perform to the best of our abilities
3. The magnitude of the responsibility of our profession (patient's lives and livelihood)
4. Financial situations
5. Electronic medical records
6. Being under constant scrutiny, with the potential for lawsuits always looming
7. Time constraints
8. Increasing non-medical responsibilities
9. Decreased autonomy
10. A relentless expectation of perfection from ourselves and others
11. Becoming more and more restrained by rules, regulations, and expectations
12. Physical and emotional demands
13. Other factors (discussed later)

How does all this translate on a pathophysiologic level? To answer this question, we only need to look at what is affected in us that are key to performing our profession:

1. Our resiliency
2. Our coping abilities

3. Our adaptive mechanisms
4. Our cognitive abilities
5. Our skills
6. Our humanity and empathy

THE ROLE OF STRESS

Most people must deal with stress at some point in their life; however, many stressors are transient in nature. Whether they are death, financial challenges, work issues, physical ailments, marital problems, or others, most stressors demand an adaptation that is limited in period. We all know that we are not ourselves when dealing with stress, and we take that into consideration, giving leeway and offering support to those who need it. Generally speaking, and depending on the person and the stress, we usually rebound to our functional self, albeit sometimes with scars. Dealing with stress has four main factors:

1. Source
2. Length of exposure
3. Personal ability
4. Time

If we dissect personal abilities further, we see that it is dependent on our emotional, physical, and psychosocial attributes. Another key here is time, which is needed to heal and rebound. When we are not afforded these factors (for example, if clinical depression is a comorbidity), our ability to deal with stress is severely impaired. In fact, there are no guarantees that we will be able to recover.

Now, what if the source of the stress was substantial and constant? What if every day a person was exposed to stress factors that affected their personal abilities and gradually eroded them? Suppose they (or a loved one) were facing a severe chronic illness. How much of their mettle would be tested? And how much pressure would they be able to handle before they became drained emotionally, physically, and psychosocially? Or, what if they woke up every day and there were new stressors added?

As physicians, that is the very nature of our profession. We wake up early and leave work late. We constantly deal with life-and-death situations that depend on little to no margin of error. Studies have shown that the higher the acuity of care, the greater the burnout. Patients' lives are at stake, and many of us have to perform procedures that are mentally and physically demanding.

Above all, we are expected to not only control our emotions at all times, but also ensure that they do not interfere with our practice of medicine. That, in itself, is extremely difficulty, as emotional self-control has a limited capacity. Like brake pads on a vehicle, emotional self-control erodes with use and can disappear over time. Faulty brake pads can lead to an accident, and in the medical profession, an accident is a morbidity or mortality outcome. Brake pads need to be replaced if the vehicle is to remain safe, and physicians must also replenish their emotional "break pads" if we want to maintain our cognitive abilities and skills. Our reality, however, is that we are rarely afforded the time, the knowledge, or the opportunity to recharge.

This is our reality check. Since stress in a physician's life is daily, increasing, and continuous, so why do we wonder why burnout is so prevalent?

A MALIGNANT DISEASE MODEL

In medicine, a malignant disease model depends on:

1. Time (the longer the time, the more advanced and invasive it becomes)
2. Cumulative effect
3. Genetic and environmental factors
4. Stage (in general, the more advanced the stage, the harder to treat)

If we now use these to talk about burnout, we can discuss it this way:

1. Time

    Burnout starts in medical school and continues to rise throughout the career. Since most physicians practice for at least twenty to thirty years, this is the length of time that they are exposed to the same severe stress factors. What malignancy would not thrive in this time frame?

2. Cumulative effect

    We already know that physicians are exposed to increasing amounts of stress. Ask anyone in the medical field about the difference between their situation when they started practicing and their current one, and most would say that they suffer from more stressors from their work now than at any other time. The compilation of that stress is astounding.

3. Genetic and environmental factors

    By genetic factors, we are referring not to the immune system (pre-malignant and malignant genes), but our ability to cope with stress, which is rooted in genetics and learned behavior/thinking. Now, let's add the environmental factors, which physicians have identified and rated on a scale of 1 to 5, with 5 being the most important (Medscape report, 2017) [3]:

    a. Having too many bureaucratic responsibilities (5.3)
    b. Spending too many hours at work (4.7)
    c. Feeling like just another cog in the wheel (4.6)
    d. Increasing computerization of practice (4.5)
    e. Income not high enough (4.1)
    f. Too many difficult patients (4.0)
    g. Insurance issues (4.0)
    h. Maintenance of certification requirements (4.0)
    i. Lack of professional fulfillment (3.9)

---

3 Medscape lifestyle report 2017: Race and ethnicity, bias and burnout. http://www.medscape.com/features/slideshow/lifestyle/2017

j. Threat of malpractice (3.9)
k. Too many patient appointments in the day (3.9)
l. Impact of the Affordable Care Act (3.7)
m. Difficult colleague, employer or staff (3.7)
n. Compassion fatigue, difficult employer (3.5)
o. Family stress (3.1)

These environmental factors fall under three main categories—unmet expectations, lack of control, or insufficient rewards—and are the core of burnout pathophysiology. Think about the life of physicians many years ago, including how they practiced, who they answered to, and what monetary and emotional rewards they received. Think of the people who looked up to them and believed them to be noble and honorable. Now think about the current situation for physicians and how much control (or lack thereof) they have. Think about their unmet expectations when they graduate and the constant scrutiny they are under with so many issues dictating their practice. Think about their rewards on all levels.

I once had the pleasure of talking to a longtime nephrologist from San Antonio, Texas, who had retired and was working pro bono in underserved countries. He looked pained as he told me about all the problems he'd had to deal with when he was working his regular job, but his face lit up with joy when he started talking about the pro bono work; when volunteering, he made his own schedule, connected with patients and what he was doing left him feeling passionate and fulfilled. A third-generation physician, he emphasized that this was what his father and grandfather had talked about and what he had aspired to when he became a doctor. He had finally found his meaning and was living it.

4. Stage
    The more advanced the stage, the harder it is to treat. To fully appreciate this statement, we only need to compare days of severe

stress with days of mild stress. Which day is easier to cope with and recover from? It goes without saying that the more burned out we are, and the longer we stay burned out, the more difficult it is to manage it, treat it, and recover from it.

The formula is straightforward: Continuous exposure to stress that is relentless and increasing in intensity, without the time to recover and heal, leads to a pervasive existence that threatens us and our patients. Burnout is a disease that destroys our very core and shakes the foundation of who we are as professionals, as human beings, and as care providers. Therefore, it has potential catastrophic implications on life itself—our own and others'.

CHAPTER 3

The Manifestations and Impact of Burnout

• • •

"Whenever a doctor cannot do good, he must be kept from doing harm."

HIPPOCRATES

WHEN THE DISCUSSION OF BURNOUT involves non-medical professions, the effects are usually focused on the individual personally and professionally. Personally, the focus is on mind, body, and soul, as well as on interactions and relationships with others. Professionally, the focus is on productivity at work and absenteeism and presentism (how productive and efficient a person is at work). When it comes to physicians, the discussion is very similar with one exception: the involvement of human lives and their outcomes. Not only are personal value and professional value at stake, but so is humanitarian value.

How does one, then, gage the true impact of burnout? What lens do we use to see its manifestations and effects? And with what scale do we create a value system to fully quantify its effects? Answering these questions requires that we analyze the effects on physicians in all three phases: the individual as a human being (personal), the professional practicing his or her craft (professional), and the patients and families involved (humanitarian).

Burnout in the Medical Field

The profession of medicine is as delicate as it is noble. As physicians, we are in constant human interaction that has its roots in moral and ethical soil. Before we take the Hippocratic Oath, we make a personal promise to ourselves that is no less important. We vow to help others to the best of our abilities, planning to give our all each and every time, and we pledge to everyone we treat that they will get our support, knowledge, and effort so that they can trust us with their lives. In fact, medicine arose out of the *PRIMAL SYMPATHY* of man to another man. The *PRIMAL* nature of this profession explains why burnout is so detrimental: It hits us at the very core of what makes our professional and personal lives meaningful.

Those not in the medical field do not understand that feeling, so it is not surprising that physicians in particular suffer from higher burnout rates than any other profession in the United States (6). Indeed, even those working in medicine do not share all the same responsibilities or effects; a surgeon's interaction is different from a cardiologist's, an internist's is different from a dermatologist's, and so on. Consequently, the potential "mistakes" we make—the errors that we are responsible for—carry different meaning, significance, and impact. If we were to use a scale to quantify such an impact, would it not be appropriate to use one that measures aspects such as morbidity and mortality? After all, these are measuring sticks and guides for us.

Does it not follow that physicians who deal with high-acuity situations, more complex problems that require extensive interventions, and circumstances where the margin of error is minimal to nonexistent, need to be held to the highest of these standards?

This is by no means an attempt to belittle some branches of medicine. We are a team, complementary and necessary, and each of us is important in our own right. The effects of stress on some specialties is direr than on others, not for degree of importance, but for demand of the specialty with respect to the burnout risk factors. It is no wonder, then, that burnout among physicians varies in intensity and prevalence across specialties.

Several Medscape surveys have shown that burnout is most prevalent among surgeons, emergency room physicians, acute care physicians, obstetricians, oncologists, and primary care physicians. These same surveys, along with numerous research studies have also shown that severity is highest among these same specialties. It is important to note that the difference between the least burned-out specialty (dermatology, at a rate of 37 percent) and the most burned-out specialty (critical care, at a rate of 53 percent) is 16 percent. It is also important to note that the highest rates range from 49 percent to 53 percent. Therefore, no matter the specialty, almost half of all physicians are burned out. Further magnifying this point is that high-burnout specialties such as acute care, surgery, and emergency medicine all have a minimal allowed margin of error.

Let's look at this reality again. Profession A has a very narrow margin of error. Of the physicians practicing profession A, 50 percent are burned out. Burned-out physicians make more mistakes, so one in every two physicians will make errors beyond the narrow margin, which will lead to high morbidity and mortality rates. Considering that patients trust their lives and outcomes to such physicians; do we truly grasp the potential consequences?

Now let's add another factor. Of those physicians who are burned out, the level of burnout is, on average, extremely high[3]. On a scale of 1 to 5, with 5 being severely burned out, physicians rate their burnout at 4.2. Of course, the more severe the burnout, the more likely that its consequences will be suffered personally and professionally. Knowing that, can we imagine the impact it will have on our patients?

IMPACT AND MANIFESTATIONS

Burnout has been likened to a malignancy because it is progressive. Students[2] as well as residents and attendings suffer from it[3]. Further, burnout is an international problem with rates increasing across the globe[4],

2 Shanafelt T.D., Hasan O., Dyrbye L.N., Sinsky C., Satele D., Sloan J., West CP. (2015) Changes in Burnout and Satisfaction With Work-Life Balance in Physicians and the General US Working Population Between 2011 and 2014. *Mayo Clinic Proceedings*. 90(12), 1600-13.
3 Medscape lifestyle report 2017: Race and ethnicity, bias and burnout. http://www.medscape.com/features/slideshow/lifestyle/2017
4 Graham J. (2016) Why are doctors plagued by depression and suicide? A crisis comes into focus. https://www.statnews.com/2016/07/21/depression-suicide-physicians/

and it has been found to be more common in females, with over 60 percent of women physicians surveyed reporting burnout[5]. Like malignancy, it tends to go unnoticed until its manifestations can no longer be ignored.

According to studies, burnout is on the rise. In 2013, 40 percent of physicians suffered from burnout. This had increased to 51 percent in 2015, as confirmed by Dr. Shanafelt et al[2]. On a personal level, there is an increased number of suicides among physicians, with a rate of three hundred to four hundred suicides per year due to depression and burnout. 50 % of medical students are burned out and 10% have suicidal ideations which have been linked directly to burnout. Once burnout is reduced, suicidal ideations tend to decrease also[5]. Obesity, alcohol and drug abuse, and depression are also more common among burned-out physicians, and burned-out physicians suffer more problems at home with their families and friends, and in general are much less happy and satisfied as human beings.

This has led to the realization that burnout is a global problem magnified by its effects on physicians as professionals. According to a 2015 Medscape report, physicians interviewed about burnout reported reduced productivity with a decline in their work quality. Further, burnout dulled clinical skills, which in turn produced less-thorough evaluation and intervention. This same report showed burned-out physicians to be less patient (48 percent), have decreased motivation or energy (39 percent), have worsening communication and listening skills (37 percent), have withdrawal behaviors and avoidance of helping others (40 percent), develop poor attitudes (37 percent), and have decreased empathy (35 percent)[6].

The effects of burnout include poorer relationships with patients and staff. Physicians become more irritable and angry, have decreased tolerance and patience, care less about their patients, and have poor therapeutic alliance and connection with everyone around them. Other

---

5   Dyrbye L.N., Thomas M.R., Massie S., Power D.V., Eacker A., Harper W., Durning S., Moutier C., Szyldo D.W., Movotny P.J., Sloan J.A., Shanafelt T.D. (2008) Burnout and Suicial Ideation among Medical Students. *Annals of Internal Medicine*. 149, 334-41.
6   Brauser D. (2015) Impact of burnout: Clinicians speak out. *http://www.medscape.com/viewarticle/839533*

studies have demonstrated an increase in medical mistakes, higher morbidity and mortality rates, and decreased physician patient satisfaction surveys. Perhaps the best summary, however, can be found in an article in the *Archives of Surgery* published in 2009[7]. The authors summarized the effects of physician burnout on a professional and personal level as follows:

Professional level

1- Worse judgement when it comes to decision making about patient care
2- Becoming hostile towards patients and staff
3- Increasing medical errors
4- Worse outcomes for patients
5- Decreased effort and commitment to safe, productive and optimal patient care
6- Becoming disengaged

Personal level

1- Psychiatric problems (Depression, anxiety, suicide)
2- Sleep deprivation and fatigue
3- Drug and alcohol addiction
4- Broken relationships
5- Worsening marital relationships
6- Retiring early

REVISITING THE SIX COMPETENCIES

With the impact of burnout in mind, let's again consider the six competencies of the ACGME:

---

7 Balch C.M., Freischlag J.A., Shanafelt T.D.(2009) Stress and Burnout Among Surgeons: Understanding and Managing the Syndrome and Avoiding the Adverse Consequences. *Archives of Surgery.* 144(4):371-376. doi:10.1001/archsurg.2008.575

1. Professionalism
2. Interpersonal and communication skills
3. Medical knowledge
4. Practice-based learning and development
5. Patient care
6. System-based practice

This malignant existence erodes into all of these competencies. Much like the undetected cancer, burnout affects them not in an immediate and apparent way. It is a gradual wearing down of the practice of medicine through an assault on all of what it takes from us as human beings first; and as physicians second.

To highlight the effects of burnout on patient outcomes and care, one effect—decreased listening and communication skills—will be used for illustration. The following have been found to be a direct consequence of poor communication skills:

* Communication breakdowns are responsible for 85 percent of sentinel events in hospitals.[8]

Let's think about this. Burnout affects our listening and communication skills, and this one competency can lead to catastrophic outcomes that have been displayed across morbidity and mortality reports on a universal level as well. The impact does not stop at morbidity and mortality.

Burnout also affects the bottom line, being one of the reasons why physicians, clinics, and hospital systems are in the red instead of in the black. Why? Because the medical field is changing from a patient care system to a patient customer care system. With the introduction of Press-Ganey scores, HCAHPS (Hospital Consumer Assessment of Healthcare Providers and Systems) and other evaluation surveys, the most recent of

---

8 Williams M., Hevelone N., Alban R.F., Hardy J.P., Oxman D.A., Garcia E., Thorsen C., Frendl G., Rogers S.O. Jr. (2010) Measuring communication in the surgical ICU: better communication equals better care. *Journal of the American College of Surgery.*

which is MACRA (Medicare Access and CHIP Reauthorization Act), the entire payment and reimbursement systems are changing.[9] Let us take the example of MACRA.

In general, surveys are used to target public opinion on issues such as friendliness, interactions, care levels, hospital responsiveness, and communication with staff, among other things. Hospitals are rated based on these surveys, and according to these ratings, they receive reimbursement. So, in addition to morbidity and mortality, we must also consider productivity and financial outcomes. Starting in 2017, a new evaluation and monitoring approach will be used, called MACRA. Here is a part of what it states:

> MIPS eligible clinicians will be able to select the six measures from a list of over 200, 80 percent of which are tailored for specialists. At least one of the six measures must be an outcome measure or high-priority measure and one must be a cross-cutting measure. High-priority measures are related to:

- Patient outcomes,
- Appropriate use,
- Patient safety,
- Efficiency,
- Patient experience,
- Care coordination.

THE CONCEPT OF THE PENDULUM

Psychologists like to talk about the mood pendulum. They talk about the nature of our moods going from one extreme to another and every day we are at some point on the pendulous swing. Burnout is no different.

---

9 https://www.cms.gov/medicare/quality-initiatives-patient-assessment-instruments/value-based-programs/macra-mips-and-apms/macra-mips-and-apms.html

At any given time:

- burnout is a contagious malignant existence that,
- undulates between minimal to extreme,
- driven by personal, professional, emotional, psychosocial, and environmental factors.

The question for us now is, what do we do about it?

CHAPTER 4

Diagnosing Burnout – Time to Hit the Panic Button

• • •

"Sometimes you don't feel the weight of something you've been carrying until you feel the weight of its release"

AUTHOR UNKNOWN

THERE ARE MANY OBSTACLES TO diagnosing burnout among physicians and other healthcare providers: Some center around time, others fear and denial, and some around lack of knowledge and know how. Let us take a closer look. Some are common with other malignancies; others are unique to burnout.

A LOOK AT THE OBSTACLES

Fear is one of the cornerstones of denial. Cancer had been, and continues to be referred to as "the other disease" in some parts of the world. Cancer is synonymous with doom and is met with fear and an overwhelming sense of suffering and finality. As physicians, we know how difficult it is to inform patients that they have a malignancy. Sometimes, even when we inform the patients, they continue to live in denial and refuse to treat it or even acknowledge it. Burnout is no different. Not only is its physiologic effect on us cancerous in its approach and manifestations, it can have the same psychosocial effect as any malignancy.

A significant number of patients having chest pain die from a heart attack due to denial; they fear that their chest pain might be related to their heart. If we asked every healthcare provider how many times they have had a patient not seek medical care because they did not want to know that there was something wrong with them, many would answer with one word: "Countless." Whether it is heart attacks or any other serious condition, denial, and lack of wanting to know seem to prevail.

Physicians also have a condition that they do not want to acknowledge: burnout. We make the worst patients because of our perceived knowledge of the problem, because we take our health for granted, and because we are sometimes too stubborn to be humble enough to follow directions. Healthcare workers with documented heart attacks still eat unhealthy foods, and smoke! Pulmonologists and respiratory therapists smoke. And burned-out physicians still overextend themselves. Perhaps we have spent so much of our time trying to control disease that we refuse to acknowledge it can control us. Call it whatever you want, but we are a tough crowd of patients!

The second hindrance to diagnosing burnout is reluctance. Think about all the effort that has gone into accepting and treating cancer in the general population (it is a battle to this day, really). We are still putting tremendous effort into identifying and increasing human immunodeficiency virus (HIV) awareness and treatment acceptance in the general population. These are diseases with documented and well-known sequelae, so how much more difficult will it be to reach that same comprehensive understanding and appreciation of burnout, especially among physicians? We are simply reluctant to address it. Burnout is a disease of emotions. How many of us are willing to acknowledge and accept its existence in general, let alone the possibility of it inflicting us individually in particular?

The third hindrance is time. Who has time to be sick? Even more, who has time to get better—or invest in their own health? Our lives are incredibly busy already, so we're not interested in adding another burden.

In addition to the obstacles of denial, reluctance, and time, burnout diagnosis and treatment is difficult because of:

* Lack of awareness
* The fact that it is an emotional disease
* Resistance to interventions
* Perceived complexity and demands of interventions
* The nature of medical practice and the demands of medicine
* Lack of available programs
* Lack of standardized approaches
* Lack of personal readiness and know-how

The challenges involved are indeed daunting. Burnout has existed for thousands of years, but now we are under a gigantic microscope that watches our every move, marks our every mistake, analyzes our every thought, and reports our every shortcoming. For physicians, Internet-based reviews, the news and media, and public reporting of physician mistakes by medical boards are just a few of the ways we are exposed to the world. The medical field has more ways to evaluate its workers than possibly any other profession, and we have reached a point where money is made (and dispensed) through assessing opinions about us.

As a result, we not only need to be aware of burnout; we also need to acknowledge and treat it.

Overcoming the Obstacles through Testing

So, what are the best ways to treat burnout? Let us if you will follow the model of HIV. When it was first discovered, we did not know what the causative agent was. We simply defined it by its skin and lung manifestations. A few years followed before we isolated the causative virus. Then, came the tremendous step of understanding the pathophysiology, increasing awareness among the health care providers and the public, advocating for screening and testing, understanding protection and safe behaviors, and finally, searching for a treatment. With burnout, that model holds true. We must strive to do the following, now that we have identified the symptoms and the causative agents:

A- Increase awareness: By any and all approved, scientific and validated sources.

B- Detect early: Through early detection, just like with any other disease. And when is the best time to screen for burnout? At least once a year, starting in medical school. This essentially makes screening not only mandatory, but also vital to survival and a great outcome. Consider how many lives have been saved due to early detection of cancers—cervical, colon, breast, testicular, and so on. If we employed regular screenings for burnout, imagine how many people we could help by catching it in the early stages and working to treat it and prevent it from worsening. Not only would physicians and healthcare workers be positively affected, but so would those who are treated by them. Screening for burnout is rather simple. The literature has described a few simple-to-administer questionnaires that have been validated and used in research. They all follow the same format, asking a series of questions about well-being and describing some alarming signs and symptoms. The test score then determines whether burnout exists, and if it does, at what stage. The same questionnaires are also used to reassess after intervention and treatment. The most commonly used burnout screening tools are the Maslach Burnout Inventory, the Burnout Measure, and the Shirom-Melamed Burnout Measure (the latter two consider exhaustion to be the root cause of burnout). Other surveys include the Copenhagen Inventory Burnout (which breaks down burnout into three facets: work-related burnout, staff burnout, and client-related burnout), the Oldenberg Burnout Inventory (which focuses on disengagement and exhaustion), and the Bergen Burnout Inventory (which looks for cynicism, exhaustion, and inadequacy occupationally). Every screening tool has its pros and cons, though we will not dive into them in this book. Our intention is to make it known that these tools are readily available and invaluable for screening and diagnosis.

C- Acknowledgement of burnout: We have to acknowledge the presence of burnout amongst ourselves, others and in our community before we are able to fully tackle it. Burnout has to be brought to the forefront. Thankfully, this is the direction we are going to.

D- Treatment: Treatment modalities that target the causative agents, our own biases, understandings, and abilities are being actively researched and studied. The fight against burnout has to be on two fronts: Factors outside the control of the physician, and factors within his or her control.

The following chapters touch on what we, as individuals, can do to help ourselves, and others.

CHAPTER 5

The Approach to Burnout Prevention and Treatment

• • •

"Attitude is a little thing that makes a big difference"

WINSTON CHURCHILL

IN THE MID-1980s, A NEW disease was discovered. The medical community had never seen anything like it before, but suddenly people were diagnosed with two diseases that seemed to be associated with each other but not the cause of the other. Something was causing homosexual men, drug abusers, and sexually promiscuous people to develop Kaposi's sarcoma and *Pneumocystis carinii* pneumonia: HIV.

After many years and billions of dollars of research, we have finally arrived at the stage where the disease is for the most part controllable, although not curable. Nowadays people live and die *with* HIV rather than *from* HIV. This example illustrates the progression of treatment discovery of new diseases, which can be delineated in this way:

1. Identify the symptoms.
2. Identify the causative agent.
3. Identify the mode of transmission and pathophysiology.
4. Understand the treatment options.
5. Initiate first protection guidelines.

6. Study potential treatment options while researching.
7. Apply the treatment options through well-designed studies.
8. Complete the studies, generate data, and make recommendations.
9. Reassess therapies that are recommended, and make changes accordingly through population studies.
10. Continue to develop new therapies until a cure has been reached.

Now, what if we took the same approach for burnout? Looking at the algorithm above, where do you think we are with burnout at this point in the book? If you answered between step 4 and 5, you would be correct (although we are still working on steps 2 and 3).

In the research on treatment options, there are two major intervention sites that are being considered: the antecedent/factors and the individual/personal. But before we talk about them, let's look a bit more at what happens during burnout, since understanding its pathophysiology will give a better comprehension of how to treat it.

Burnout at the PIP (Physician Interaction with Patient)

Thus far, we have talked about the factors leading to burnout. Now we need to look at the effects of burnout on the PIP, or the point of contact with a patient.

Our decisions and reactions come from certain centers in our brain, specifically the prefrontal cortex or neocortex. These centers are responsible for our development of a rational approach to the problem we are analyzing; they help us think. When our minds are clear, we think to the best of our abilities. But what about when our minds are clouded? What happens to our decision-making abilities then?

Self-control—or the process of maintaining an emotionally neutral or positive position so that we can make an unbiased, well-thought-out decision—is a finite ability. The neocortex sits atop the midbrain, which makes decisions based on emotional, not rational, processes. As long as the midbrain, specifically the amygdala, is kept in check, we are able to use our neocortex and will not be "hijacked" by the amygdala. The process of burnout is the loss of that neocortex function and the hijacking of our decision-making process by an angry, irritable, or negatively charged amygdala.

We can again use the analogy of brake pads, with self-control. If we use them continuously—without changing them or recharging—they will erode until they no longer work, and then we will have an accident. Similarly, if we don't give our self-control abilities a break and let them revitalize, we will lose that self-control and end up with a decision made by the amygdala due to the neocortex being burned out. In the medical field, this translates to us and our patient crashing. (The result of that process is demonstrated below in a set of tables that illustrate how we migrate from the left [high] side of the table to the right [low] side.)

Let's now review what is needed to make a clear decision and be able to fully comprehend the patient and the problem at hand. In the tables below, the left side is what is needed to get the best PIP outcome, while the right side is what happens when we are burned out. These descriptions are from Multi Health Systems in their research on the Emotional Quotient Inventory (EQi, 2.0)[10]. Using them, consider making a clinical judgment while experiencing the emotions on the left side and then on the right. Compare the potential outcomes, which not only apply to the patient but also to us and our daily life. Going back to the example of self-control being finite, similar to brake pads, notice how the transformation happens[10].

Impulse Control

High	Low
Composed	Explosive
Patient	Unpredictable
Ability to delay or resist an impulse	Reactive
High tolerance to frustration	Easily frustrated
	Aggressive

---

10 Stein S.J., Book H.E. (2011) The EQ Edge: Emotional Intelligence and Your Success Paperback. Jossey-Bass. 3rd Edition. ISBN-10: 0470681616

Problem Solving

High	Low
Gathers information first, uses pros and cons when permitted	Jumps into solutions
Can identify and solve problems	Flies by the seats of the pants
Uses a systematic approach	Uses unstructured strategy
Can apply emotional information to help	
Can draw on past experiences	

Reality Testing

High	Low
Tuned into environment	Tuned out
Can assess life situations fairly accurately	Unrealistic
Grounded	Disconnected
Objective	Easily swayed

Empathy

High	Low
Sensitive to feelings of others	Difficulty understanding people's feelings
Able to put self in other's shoes	Difficulty relating to others
Anticipates other's reactions	Surprised by other's reactions
Picks up on social cues	Misreads social cues

Interpersonal Relationships

High	Low
Ability to establish mutually satisfying relationships	Is not comfortable with intimacy

Ability to give and take affection and intimacy	Not giving
Maintains relationships over time	Not interested in relationships
Looks positively at social change	Not able to share feelings
Feels at ease in social situations	Loner and standoffish

COMBATTING BURNOUT

Two of the key components in combating burnout, preventing it, and treating it are wellness and emotional intelligence. In the following chapters, we will be discussing these two and demonstrating the inherent link between our ability to practice medicine, burnout, self-healing, wellness, and emotional intelligence. Here is the outline (which will be followed by the rationale):

1. We know we need our intelligence quotient (IQ) and emotional quotient (EQ) to best practice medicine.
2. We also know that the factors causing burnout affect both our IQ and EQ.
3. Further, we know that with EQ, we have adequate "optics" to self-diagnose ourselves and understand where we are on the pendulum of burnout.
4. We also know that our EQ abilities are instrumental in fighting burnout.
5. We know that we need wellness to fortify our EQ and in turn IQ, with the effects noticeable in the art and science of practicing medicine.

THE ANTECEDENT/FACTORS SITE

While we know there are many external factors that lead to physician burnout and ultimately push us to the "low" side of our abilities, and while physicians have spoken about these factors, few know what to do about them. Through conversations with the American College of Physicians, the ACGME, the National Academy of Sciences, the Association for Hospital Medical Education, and the Association of American Medical Colleges, there is a consensus that interventions need to happen on a local, institutional, national, and international stage. These entities have therefore joined forces, but the approach may have been already outlined by Dr. Shanafelt and his group at the Mayo Clinic. The question that remains is how to implement their guidelines[11].

In April 2016, Dr. Shanafelt published a comprehensive approach that outlined areas of potential interventions. He targeted five major areas: workload, efficiency, control over work/autonomy, work–life integration, and meaning at work. Again, the points of intervention were divided into individual, work unit, organization, and national factors. The aspects targeted included productivity expectations, reimbursement, and structure[11].

He proposed increasing the efficiency and use of allied health professionals at a work unit level, stressing increasing efficiency and streamlining the patient experience while calling for more staff and peer support along with systems and electronic health record support. He suggested increasing the degree of flexibility in scheduling and policy development, and finally, a call was made to change organizational culture, leadership, and values, thus improving, evolving, and integrating more supervisory roles for physicians and making them part of the decision-processing team. Also of importance was matching talent to areas of practice and interest, with increasing opportunities for education, leadership, and research. It is beyond this book to talk

---

11 Shanafelt T.D., Mungo M., Schmitgen J., Storz K.A., Reeves D., Hayes S.N., Sloan J.A., Swensen S.J., Buskirk S.J. (2016) Longitudinal Study Evaluating the Association Between Physician Burnout and Changes in Professional Work Effort. *Mayo Clinic Proceedings.* 91(4), 422-31

about the external risk factors. It is our goal to focus on the individual factors.

THE PERSONAL/INDIVIDUAL SITE

On a personal/individual level, Dr. Shanafelt proposed that physicians need to be able to accumulate experience and be able to prioritize. They also must improve their personal efficiency, have the willingness to delegate, develop the ability to say no, be able to prioritize, be assertive, and develop a balance between work and life. Further, they need to improve their own self-awareness and be able to integrate their work–life balance while maintaining satisfaction in their work, happiness in their personal life.

While societies and academia debate how to exactly achieve the necessary changes to be implemented at the outside-factors levels, the focus here will be on how to achieve the personal requirements to combat burnout. In a personal interview with the American Medical Association, and echoed by other societies, 80 percent of burnout is believed to be due to antecedent factors. Even if that is the case, individual-level factors must also be addressed, since the fight against burnout starts from within. If we are able to "vaccinate", fortify and enhance our innate abilities to fight burnout, then we are able to achieve a few simultaneous important goals:

A- We take control of our lives and burnout (remember lack of control is one risk factor for burnout).

B- We shift the focus to what we are able to do on an individual level and make us more resilient, focused and "stronger". When we are in that state, we are better equipped and able to fight the antecedent factors.

C- We personalize our approach. What works for one of us does not work for the others. The foundations of change that are needed are universal, as you will discover. The implementations are as unique as our own DNA.

D- It is rewarding. As healthcare providers, we want to be able to solve the problem. We are wired to diagnose and treat. It provides us with great positive energy when we are able to identify a disease and conquer it, so to speak. Imagine you are diagnosed with burnout, but now you possess your own tools to fight it. The innate boost it provides you is tremendous.

E- We have given multiple workshops and presentations on burnout. We can tell you from experience that the degree of relief and strength participants feel once they understand, implement, and see results are palpable and reproducible. Imagine giving your patient power and control over his or her cancer! It strikes the very core of what makes malignancy such a horrible disease: its ability to control and slowly erode our lives with what seemingly feels at times a lost battle, a hopeless fight, and a complete surrender to the inevitable.

F- While we wait for governments and institutions to implement changes, we can take immediate action on ourselves. This is what this book is all about. It is to introduce us to the ways that we can use to immediately push back against burnout. This malignancy is not waiting on us. Which malignancy does?

In 2011, Dr. Shanafelt summarized and echoed findings from multiple references and resources. He summed that all physicians "deal with stressful times in their personal and professional life and must cultivate habits of personal renewal, emotional self-awareness, connection with colleagues, adequate support systems, and the ability to find meaning in work to combat these challenges".[12] What we must determine now is how to do that. How do we achieve the individual goals and "cultivate habits of personal renewal, emotional self-awareness, connection with colleagues, adequate support systems, and the ability to find meaning in work to combat these challenges"?

The answer involves two things: wellness and emotional intelligence.

---

12 Balch C.M., Shanafelt T. (2011) Combating stress and burnout in surgical practice: a review. *Thoracic Surgery Clinics*, 21(3), 417-30.

CHAPTER 6

Emotional Intelligence, the Practice of Medicine and Burnout

• • •

"Know thyself"

Socrates

Since burnout is a disease of emotions, logic suggests that the key to preventing and treating burnout lies in the emotional realm.

All physicians are familiar with IQ, which is a measure of cognitive abilities that reflects our book smarts and mental abilities. As practicing physicians, IQ is responsible for no more than 25 percent of our ability to perform our job[13]. In fact, IQ is dependent on another type of intelligence: emotional intelligence (EI).

According to psychologist Dr. Daniel Goleman, EI is "the capacity for recognizing our own feelings and those of others, for motivating ourselves, for managing emotions well in ourselves and in our relationships." It refers to a set of abilities that are inherent, measurable, and, perhaps most important of all, modifiable. These abilities help us perceive, understand, regulate, and manage our own emotions as well as those of others, providing us

---

13   Goleman D. (2002). Primal Leadership. Harvard Business Press 2002.

with the necessary tools to be aware of and better manage ourselves and others. Review of the literature shows a marked increase in the study and possible application the concept of EI in the field of medicine.

There are fifteen realms of emotional intelligence assessed in the EQi, 2.0 by Multi Health Systems, and are illustrated in the diagram below. These will be discussed in greater detail.

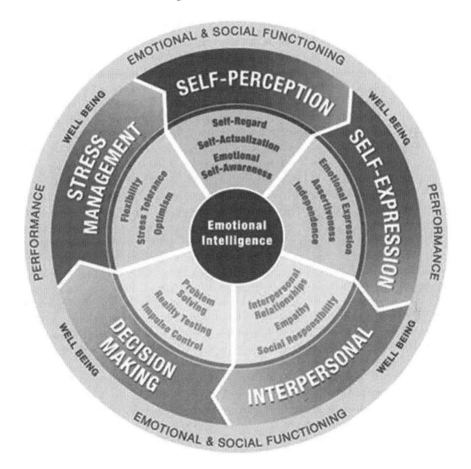

The definitions/relevance of each EQ realm and competency are as follows:

1. Self-Perception Realm:
   a. Emotional self-awareness: The ability to recognize your feelings, understand their differences, where they come from and how they impact others.
   b. Self-regard: Your confidence and the ability to accept and respect yourself.
   c. Self-actualization: The ability to realize your true potential and strive to reach it.

   This cluster helps answer the following questions:
   * How aware am I of how my emotions affect myself and others?
   * How confident am I?
   * Am I constantly trying to improve?

2. Self-Expression Realm:
   a. Emotional expression: The ability to openly and appropriately expressing your feelings verbally and nonverbally.
   b. Independence: The ability to stand on one's own two feet and accept responsibility.
   c. Assertiveness: The ability to express feelings, beliefs, and thoughts openly, and to stand up for personal rights.

   This cluster will help answer the following questions:
   * Can I speak appropriately about the uncomfortable experiences and emotions that arise during the work day?
   * Can I make decisions autonomously?
   * Can I defend my points of view in a non-offensive manner?

3. Interpersonal Realm:
   a. Interpersonal relationships: The ability to give and take with others, in a compassionate way that builds trust
   b. Empathy: The ability to tune in to how and what people feel and think, and why they feel and think the way they do.
   c. Social responsibility: The desire and willingness to contribute positively to society and your environment by acting

responsibly, guided by your conscience, and fulfilled by the benefit of others.

This cluster will help answer the following questions:

* Do patients and co-workers trust and want to work with me?
* Do they feel that I really get them and their concerns?
* Am I a helpful member of the community?

4. Decision Making Realm:

   a. Reality testing: Seeing objectively, not clouded with emotions or biases. A measure of pragmatism, adequacy of perception, and authentic ideas and thoughts.

   b. Problem solving: The ability to solve problems where emotions are involved, by understanding those emotions and not just the problem. It is directly related to the desire to confront problems, not avoid them, and do your best.

   c. Impulse control: Ability to avoid rash or impulsive decisions, minimizing emotional outcomes and focusing on rational ones.

   This cluster will help answer the following questions:

   * Can I stay objective and see the situation as it is?
   * Can I find good solutions when my emotions are hijacked?
   * Am I able to manage my impulses and reactions in what I say and do?

5. Stress Management Realm:

   a. Flexibility: The ability to detect changing situations and conditions and adjust your thoughts, emotions and behavior accordingly navigating the sometimes-rough waters of the medical field, both patient-wise and system-wise.

   b. Stress tolerance: Dealing with stress, making the most of stress, and being optimistic.

   c. Optimism: A *realistic*, positive outlook on life even in the darkest of times.

This cluster will help answer the following questions:

* How adaptable am I?
* How much stress can I handle?
* What is my attitude when there are difficult circumstances?

Reviewing the literature shows a tremendous link between the practice of medicine and our emotional intelligence. EI is measured through a series of questions that produce an EQ score or an emotional quotient just like an intelligence quotient. That score reflects our performance in the different realms and shows where we are competent and where we need development. For example, one may have a strong self-awareness but lack impulse control and communication abilities. The translation, as far as the physician–patient interaction, is a confident physician who cannot communicate and is emotionally labile and more prone to mistakes because of poor impulse control. How many of us are like that or know someone who is?

EI may be the missing link between the reality of burnout in our profession and the discovery of its cure. As we dig deeper into this relationship, let's review some of what the literature has already shown with respect to EI and the practice of medicine.

Some EI Statistics

1. Research has shown promise in advocating the use of EI-based education systems to develop and improve the art of professional development and communication skills[14].
2. A study of 2,800 physician "star performers" showed that 75 percent of a high-achiever's success is a function of emotional intelligence; only 25 percent of success reflects technical competency.
3. Unlike IQ, which is generally fixed at a certain age …
   a. EI competencies can be learned.
   b. EQ skills can be developed.

---

14 Cherry, M.G., Fletcher, I., O'Sullivan, H., Dornan, T. (2014) Emotional intelligence in medical education: a critical review. *Medical Education*. 48(5), 468-78.

    c. One can develop emotional intelligence.

    d. One can "rewire" their responses to stress and emotions.

    e. One can change how they think about stress and deal with emotions.

    f. One can learn to alter behavior to co-workers.

    g. One can learn to make better decisions.

4. It has been shown that paying closer attention to and understanding a patient's emotional cues, having a better awareness of the patient's emotional status, and communicating with more empathy lead to a positive impact on both the physician–patient relationship and personal physician growth, development, and well-being[15].

5. EQ has reliable and valid assessment tools[16].

6. The foundations of EI are in effective leadership success and performance, not the morality of right or wrong. Studies have proposed that EI abilities should be able to provide specific curricula, which, if successfully learned by residents and students, and effectively taught by faculty, would account for improved professionalism in trainees. This is possible through approaches and skills not currently present in the way curricula are taught currently[17].

7. Weng et al., in 2011, advocated the need for creating programs that teach and promote EI for medical professionals. They acknowledged the potential positive effects of such programs on physician and patient satisfaction[18].

15 Satterfield, J., Swenson, S., Rabow, M. (2009) Emotional Intelligence in Internal Medicine Residents: Educational Implications for Clinical Performance and Burnout. *Annals of Behavioral Science and Medical Education.* 14(2), 65-68.

16 Ciarrochi JV, Chan AYC, Caputi P. (2000) A critical evaluation of the emotional intelligence construct. *Personality and Individual Differences.* 28:539–561.

17 Taylor, C., Farver, C., Stoller, J.K. (2011) Perspective: Can emotional intelligence training serve as an alternative approach to teaching professionalism to residents? *Academic Medicine.* 86(12), 1551-4.

18 Weng H.C., Hung C.M., Liu Y.T., Cheng Y.J., Chang C.C., Huang C.K. (2011) Associations between emotional intelligence and doctor burnout, job satisfaction and patient satisfaction. *Medical Education.* 45, 835-42.

8. Training in EI is needed in undergraduate and graduate medical education[19].

9. The practice of medicine, as well as the interaction of physicians with the patients, healthcare organizations, government, and corporate medicine necessitate the development of a new skill that is dependent on physicians' ability to collaborate care. The inability for collaboration will produce stress and further burnout among physicians. This new ability and the new demands, which are not taught in medical schools or in graduate medical education, are dependent on core competencies that are measured, studied, and improved by EI. The need to develop programs that target these new roles among physicians using EI is evident and necessary[20].

10. Studies have shown that EQ is able to predict academic success. Further, it can also predict multicultural counseling knowledge, show who has empathy and optimism[21], identify people with social skills, and identify individuals who have the ability to problem solve effectively[22].

11. EQ may be able to discover an important skill set that predicts professional and personal outcomes, which is not seen by available and currently used intelligence and achievement tests[23].

19 Stoller J.K., Taylor C.A., Farver C.F.(2013) Emotional intelligence competencies provide a developmental curriculum for medical training. *Medical Teacher.* 35(3), 243-7.

20 Mintz L.J., Stoller J.K. (2014) A systematic review of physician leadership and emotional intelligence. *Journal of Graduate Medical Education.* 6(1), 21-31.

21 Constantine M.G., Gainor K.A. (2001) Emotional intelligence and empathy: Their relation to multicultural counseling knowledge and awareness. *Professional School of Counseling.* 5:131–137.

22 Schutte N.S., Schuettpelz E., Malouff J.M. (2001) Emotional intelligence and task performance. *Imagination, Cognition, and Personality.* 20:347–354.

23 McManus IC, Smithers E, Partridge P, Keeling A, Fleming PR. (2003) A levels and intelligence as predictors of medical careers in UK doctors: 20 year prospective study. *British Medical Journal.* 327:139–142.

12. Research has shown promise in advocating the use of EI-based education systems to develop and improve the art of professional development and communication skills[24].

13. The foundations of EI are in effective leadership success and performance, not the morality of right or wrong. Studies have proposed that EI abilities should be able to provide specific curricula, which, if successfully learned by residents and students, and effectively taught by faculty, would account for improved professionalism in trainees. This is possible through ways and properties not currently present in the way curricula are taught currently[25].

14. Weng et al., in 2011, advocated the need for creating programs that teach and promote EI for medical professionals. They acknowledged the potential positive effects of such programs on physician and patient satisfaction[18].

15. Training in EI is needed in undergraduate and graduate medical education[20].

16. Using coaching techniques that focus on improving self-awareness, self-care, self-compassion, and boundary setting have led to behavioral changes among physicians and improved patient care[26].

17. Medical schools have been urged to address communication and interpersonal skills using EI[27].

18. In a critical review of the literature performed by Arora et al. in 2010[28], the authors identified a total of 485 articles that have looked at EI in medicine. Through rigorous review criteria that focused

---

24 Cherry, M.G., Fletcher, I., O'Sullivan, H., Dornan, T. (2014) Emotional intelligence in medical education: a critical review. *Medical Education*. 48(5), 468-78.

25 Taylor, C., Farver, C., Stoller, J.K. (2011) Perspective: Can emotional intelligence training serve as an alternative approach to teaching professionalism to residents? *Academic Medicine*. 86(12), 1551-4.

26 Schneider S., Kingslover K., Rosdahl J. (2014) Physician coaching to enhance well-being: a qualitative analysis of a pilot intervention. *Explore*. 10(6):372-9.

27 Webb A.R., Young R.A., Baumer J.G. (2010) Emotional Intelligence and the ACGME competencies. *Journal of Graduate Medical Education*. 508-12.

28 Arora S., Ashrafian H., Davis R., Athansiou T., Darzi A., Sevdalis N.(2010) Emotional intelligence in medicine: a systematic review through the context of the ACGME competencies. Medical Education. 44, 749-764.

on scientific merit and commonality of purpose and approaches, they narrowed their source to 16 articles. In their review, they looked at EI as a concept and an ability. The authors discussed the importance of EI with respect to the six core competencies of the ACGME. They noted the EI is inherently linked to empathy, effective communication, leadership, stress management, teamwork, and academic performance. EI's inherent characteristics are such that they warrant further studies and programs aimed at cultivating them and training medical professionals in them. The problem is the lack of uniform approaches based on concrete evidence derived from studies and data-driven research. The authors conclude that the importance of EI cannot be understated and that it is crucial to learn how to effectively teach it and apply it to all medical personnel at all levels.

The interventions in this field have begun. A survey by Dean Stephen Klasko, M.D., M.B.A., Dean of University of South Florida College of Medicine and CEO of USF Health found:

- "60% of physicians practicing three years or less were 'frustrated' that they did not learn what they most needed in practice. They learned microbiology and anatomy, cardiology, and internal medicine. But they did not learn how to creatively embrace change, effectively communicate or collaboratively negotiate."
- 2011, USF Health is leading change with the SELECT program— Scholarly Excellence, Leadership Experiences, and Collaborative Training.
- MCAT's in 2015 to include:
  - Social psychological, social science, and communication, humanistic questions
  - Fundamental Attribution Theory
  - A move toward inclusion of EI Competencies

As the link is being established between EI and the practice of medicine, another link, no less important, has been documented between EI and burnout. What we know so far can be summarized as follows.

From 2010 to 2014, we have seen an explosion of reviews and studies on EI in the field of medicine, looking at physician burnout in particular. There seems to be a more focused approach to linking the concepts of EI and their relevance on burnout. The issue of burnout has taken an important aspect of its own for its documented effects on physician well-being, physician performance, physician satisfaction, patient satisfaction, risk reduction, and improved outcomes.

Research on physicians and EQ/EI shows physicians to have lower-than-average scores (while also having above-average IQ scores). In general, physicians are highly technical in their respective areas but seem to lack communication skills, empathy, and the intercommunication skills needed to provide exceptional patient-centered medical practice[29]. Review of the literature also shows that EI is paramount to providing healthcare professionals the necessary skills to help them successfully manage the many roles they need to play (supporters, friends and colleagues, experts and partners, supervisors and mentors). Research also shows that these skills are often not taught, not the focus of educational programs, and not the focus of training forums or courses[30].

Finally, there is another reason why having a high EQ is extremely important in the practice of medicine: "optics."

THE CONCEPT OF OPTICS

Optics refers to the ability to be able to read and understand instruments, like doing so in a cockpit to fly a plane. Without the optics, the pilot would be lost and most likely crash and burn. Likewise, without optics, we cannot evaluate/see/diagnose/recognize burnout.

---

29 Wagner, P., Moseley, G., Grant, M., Gore, J., Owens, C. (2002) Physicians' emotional intelligence and patient satisfaction. *Family Medicine.* 34(10), 750-54.

30 Stein, S., Book, H. (2011) *The EQ edge: Emotional intelligence and your success.* 3rd ed. Mississauga, Ont. Jossey-Bass.

Since our body communicates with us all the time, the question raised is how do we recognize the signs and symptoms of burnout? How do we self-diagnose ourselves? With a broken leg, the first sign is pain, never mind the swelling and discoloration. In this case, physical pain is what is perceived by the body as the "optical" signal that something is wrong, so we don't bear weight on that leg. All people recognize physical pain; it is one of the first sensations we encounter after we come into this world. I doubt anyone would consider standing on a broken leg for minutes, let alone hours, to operate. We can't run a clinic, work in the emergency room, and be in the endoscopy suite unless some form of pain intervention happens. Whether it is a cast, a boot, or otherwise, we would need reduced pain and comfort to perform our duties.

The same is true when it comes to burnout: we need reduced pain and comfort to perform our duties. And how does the body talk to us when we are burned out? We've already discussed the signs and symptoms of burnout, but the problem often lies not in those, but in our ability to perceive, recognize, understand, and react to them. This is where emotional intelligence is even more important.

If we are emotionally intelligent about ourselves, then we have the ability to read and understand the optics of burnout's manifestations on our emotional, physical, and psychosocial states. Research has shown that the body perceives pain as pain, no matter whether the source is physical, social, or emotional; the perception is still pain[31]. If it is unthinkable to practice medicine on a broken leg without some form of intervention, how would it be possible to practice medicine with broken emotions and burnout without intervention?

If we discover that a certain malignancy (burnout) affects a certain type of tissue (emotions), and if we also discover that this malignancy operates in such a way to disrupt communication among the cells of this tissue and interferes with their abilities to perform their job (loss

31 Eisenberger NI. Why rejection hurts: what social neuroscience has revealed about the brain's response to social rejection. In: Decety J, Cacioppo J, editors. *The Handbook of Social Neuroscience*. New York, NY: Oxford. University Press; 2011:109Y27.

of emotional abilities and intelligence), then how do we stop this malignancy from working the way it does? When and where do we treat? At which level should the treatment work, and what are the target areas of treatment? And finally, what chemotherapeutic agent and delivery system should be used?

Being emotionally intelligent translates to improved ability of performing in the medical profession and being able to detect and combat burnout. It follows, then, that programs need to be implemented to target emotional intelligence to improve and fortify it.

We know that EI is linked to medical practice and is essential for a positive physician–patient interaction. We also know that EQ and IQ are affected negatively by burnout, which is an escalating consequence of practicing medicine. Further, we now know that implementing programs or approaches that serve to increase and fortify EQ will help in combating burnout and improving the practice of medicine. Developing these programs relies on practices and philosophies that are based in wellness and emotional intelligence training.

In their efforts to try to create a new burnout questionnaire screening tool, Moreno-Jimenez et al. (2012) studied the impact of burnout on the physician on several fronts[32]. Their research led them to the following conclusion:

---

32 Moreno-Jiménez B., Barbaranelli C., Herrer MG., Hernández EG. (2012) The physician burnout questionnaire: A new definition and measure. *TPM - Testing, Psychometrics, Methodology in Applied Psychology, 19*(4), 325-344. DOI: 10.4473/TPM19.4.6.

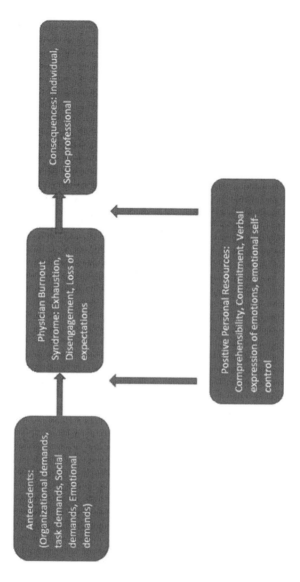

It is in the positive personal resources that we inject EI. In the up-coming chapters, we will look in more detail at these programs from an emotional intelligence and a wellness perspective.

CHAPTER 7

Emotional Intelligence and the Practice of Medicine

• • •

*"Illustrious doctors might have graduated from
books, but books made not a single physician"*

SIR WILLIAM OSLER QUOTING PARACELSUS

THE TERM *SOCIAL INTELLIGENCE* WAS first used by psychologist Edward Thorndike in 1920. Decades later, in 1983, another psychologist, Howard Gardner, wrote about seven types of intelligences in *Frames of Mind*[33]. Two of the seven types were intrapersonal intelligence and interpersonal intelligence, the core of today's EI models.

In 1985, Dr. Reuven Bar-On first coined the term *emotional quotient,* or EQ[34]. He saw EQ as a set of emotional and social skills that influence the way we:

1. Perceive and express ourselves
2. Develop and maintain social relationships
3. Cope with challenges
4. Use emotional information in an effective and meaningful way.

---

33 Gardner H. (1983) *Frames of Mind*. Basic Books. Underlining and Notation edition (1983).
34 EQi 2.0 User's Handbook 2011, Toronto Canada: Multi Health System.

In 1990, Salovey and Mayer first used the term *emotional intelligence* in a research paper, stating that "our framework for emotional intelligence, is a set of skills hypothesized to contribute to the accurate appraisal and expression of emotion in oneself and in others, the effective regulation of emotion in self and others, and the use of feelings to motivate, plan and achieve in one's life". [35]

Dr. Goleman then popularized the term with his books *Emotional Intelligence* (1995)[36] and *Working with Emotional Intelligence* (2000)[37]. The simple definition we have adopted for emotional intelligence is, understanding and managing yourself and understanding and managing others.

THE EI FORMULA: MOMENT MASTERY (PIP)

Emotional intelligence has been explained as "strategic intelligence," a term that resonated with the military when this model was presented. How do we "master the moment" with great decision making and communication? We must be particularly aware of the input from ourselves and others so our output is exceptional.

The formula we use for the mathematically minded is:

$$\text{Empathy (E)} * \text{Insight (I)} * \text{Clarity (C)} = \text{Top 10 \% Performance}$$
$$E*I*C = \text{Top 10\%}$$

Empathy includes an individual's observable signs as well as invisible feelings. We use this information or input to make decisions and adjustments, like during a typical day of seeing patients. The more clarity and

35 Salovey P., Mayer J. D. (1990). Emotional intelligence. *Imagination, Cognition, and Personality*. 9, 185-211. doi:0.2190/DUGG-P24E-52WK-6CDG.

36 Goleman D. (1995) *Emotional intelligence: Why it can matter more than IQ*. Bloomsbury; 12.2.1995 edition.

37 Goleman D. (2000) *Working with Emotional Intelligence*. Bantam; Reprint edition.

knowledge we have about these signs, the less potential risks and better decisions or output we will make. Spending time with patients and co-workers to truly understand them incorporates listening carefully, asking follow-up questions, and respecting their feelings and opinions.

The *insight* part of the equation is also invisible and often overlooked as means of obtaining information (or input) and knowledge. The ability to know our biases, strengths, and weaknesses, and emotional triggers that lower our impulse control and impair communication is vital to optimal patient interactions and medical decision making.

When we are interacting with others—patients and co-workers—what emotional intelligence are we exhibiting? What is our external awareness, and can we make the appropriate adjustments? And what is our internal awareness, and can we make the appropriate adjustments?

In 1991, Dr. Goleman collaborated with his colleague Dr. Richard Boyatzis and the Hay Group to come up with the Emotional Competence Inventory (ECI). One version has eighteen competencies and another has twelve competencies, and both are a 360-degree assessment. A wealth of research on the ECI competencies has been promoted by the Hay Group over the last thirty years, based on four clusters areas: Understanding Yourself, Managing Yourself, Understanding Others, and Managing Others. Both the EQ-i and ECI are considered a mixed focus on both traits and abilities.

The last test we will look at is more of an abilities measure: the Mayer-Salovey-Caruso Emotional Intelligence Test, or MSCEIT. It includes the ability to label emotions, understand the relationships between words and feelings, distinguish between authentic and non-authentic emotional expressions, and manage emotions by strengthening positive and reducing negative ones.

Measuring EQ is important, but more essential is having a development plan to enhance strengths and minimize weaknesses. So how do we do that? By understanding the five realms of emotional intelligence with their competencies. Our abilities—our emotional intelligence—can be scientifically measured in a valid and reliable methodology, and that is significant because when something is measurable, it is quantifiable, observable, and, perhaps most important of all, modifiable.

Emotional Intelligence's Main Pillars

There are two main pillars of emotional intelligence: The first is its application and relevance to burnout, and the second is its ability to be modified and enhanced to produce change in one's self that leads to a decrease in burnout rates and severities, and ultimately better clinical outcomes. To illustrate this, let's focus on one of the ACGME competencies: communication skills.

Measuring the EQ of a physician will highlight their strengths and weaknesses in areas that are needed for better communication skills. One of these areas is the realm of self-expression. Physicians who are inferior communicators score poorly in the self-expression realm. The relevance of the EQ test is that it outlines these deficiencies and points them out in a quantifiable manner. Once deficiencies are identified, intervention processes follow.

The intervention process has seven steps:

1. Assess the physician's EQ competencies.
2. Decide which competencies are best to improve and do more of, considering the physician's results, position, and ACGME competencies.
3. Identify key tools to improve these EQ competencies.
4. Create a plan for improvement.
5. Practice these competencies.
6. Reevaluate competency level.
7. Make a follow-up plan to maintain the progress.

Emotional intelligence can be learned and improved, unlike IQ, which is static. Interventions are less developed than the assessment of EQ at this point. Like medical training, there is a process to becoming skilled in emotional intelligence competencies.

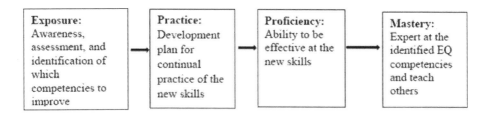

Exposure: Awareness, assessment, and identification of which competencies to improve	→	Practice: Development plan for continual practice of the new skills	→	Proficiency: Ability to be effective at the new skills	→	Mastery: Expert at the identified EQ competencies and teach others

We will now go more into depth about the EQ-i 2.0. Both competencies and clusters will be explored along with some case studies to help elucidate the interplay and balance of the competencies. All of these work together in a systematic way, like the body, to impact emotional and social functioning and overall performance. Some competencies may need to be improved, or "dialed up," and some competencies may need to be "dialed down." The result can be a prevention of burnout and an intervention to lessen physician burnout and dissatisfaction. Presented here is an introductory overview.

15 EQ-i^{2.0} Scales and Subscales

Self-Perception
- Self-Regard
- Self-Actualization
- Emotional Self-Awareness

Self-Expression
- Emotional Expression
- Assertiveness
- Independence

Interpersonal
- Interpersonal Relationships
- Empathy
- Social Responsibility

Decision Making
- Problem Solving
- Reality Testing
- Impulse Control

Stress Management
- Flexibility
- Stress Tolerance
- Optimism

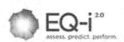

34

As you look at the competencies above, which are the top five that you think are most important for you to excel at for reducing risks?

SELF-PERCEPTION CLUSTER

Our character is basically a composite of our habits.
Because they are consistent, often unconscious patterns,
they constantly, daily, express our character.

—STEPHEN COVEY

The self-perception cluster involves the inner self and is made up of self-regard, self-actualization, and emotional self-awareness. It is "designed to assess feelings of inner strength and confidence, persistence in the pursuit of personally relevant and meaningful goals while understanding what, when, why and how different emotions impact thoughts and actions[34]." This translates to the following questions:

* How confident am I?
* Am I constantly trying to get better?
* How aware am I of how my emotions affect me and others?

This cluster is the most important place to start and to master. Knowing your self well gives you information and data that not only helps manage yourself, but also shows you what to change, adjust, or manage. It incorporates the insight and clarity part of our top 10 percent equation. As Socrates said, "The unexamined life is not worth living." And according to Benjamin Franklin, "There are three things extremely hard: steel, a diamond, and to know one's self."

Self-regard is knowing and accepting your strengths, and is often associated with self-confidence. Do you accept yourself and feel good about yourself?

Self-actualization is striving to be better, being driven to achieve, being self-motivated, and living a meaningful life. Self-improvement and continuous learning are examples of this competency.

Emotional self-awareness is being knowledgeable about your emotions, understanding which ones contribute to your performing at peak, which ones get in your way, how your emotions influence others, and how your emotions impact your decision making. We all have blind spots; it's just that good leaders and top performers have fewer of them.

In a *Forbes* magazine article, a study of 6,977 self-assessments from professionals at 486 publicly traded companies identified the "blind spots"—defined disparities between self-reported skills and peer ratings—present. They found that "poor performing companies' employees were 79 percent more likely to have low overall self-awareness than those at firms with robust return on revenue. Stock performance was tracked over thirty months, from July 2010 through January 2013. During that period the companies with the greater percentage of self-aware employees consistently outperformed those with a lower percentage". [38]

In 2010, the Hay Group found leaders with higher self-awareness also had heightening of many of the other EI/EQ competencies. This was to a degree more than they expected.[39]

SELF-EXPRESSION CLUSTER

The single biggest problem in communication is the illusion that it has taken place."

GEORGE BERNARD SHAW

---

38 https://www.kornferry.com/institute/647-a-better-return-on-self-awareness
39 https://atrium.haygroup.com/downloads/marketingps/nz/ESCI_research_findings_2010.pdf

This self-expression cluster involves the outward expressions or action components of the internal perceptions from the cluster above—in other words, openly expressing thoughts and feelings in a constructive way. It includes emotional expression, assertiveness, and independence. This translates to the following questions:

* Can I speak appropriately about the uncomfortable experiences and emotions that arise during the workday?
* Can I defend my points of view in a non-offensive manner?
* Can I make decisions autonomously?

Emotional expression is openly expressing your feelings verbally and non-verbally. Given the variety of emotions experienced during the day, from anger to disappointment to sadness and regret, can you express these effectively so people know what is happening for you?

Assertiveness is expressing your opinions and recommendations, and defending your personal rights in an appropriate and inoffensive manner.

Independence is making decisions without dependency on others and making the appropriate call autonomously.

The ACGME competencies of communication, interpersonal skills, and patient care will be impacted by a professional who scores high in these self-expression competencies.

INTERPERSONAL CLUSTER

> *So much of what we call management consists in*
> *making it difficult for people to work.*

—PETER DRUCKER

The interpersonal cluster involves developing good relations based on trust and compassion. It is understanding others and showing concern for the others. This cluster includes interpersonal relations, empathy, and social responsibilities. This translates to the following questions:

* Do patients and co-workers trust and want to work with me?
* Do they feel that I really get them and their concerns?
* Am I a helpful member of the community?

Interpersonal relationships is your ability to make good relationships, and have people want to confide in you and feel comfortable talking to you about their issues. An important part of this competency would be your bedside manner.

Empathy is being sensitive to others' feelings and being able to anticipate their reactions.

Social Responsibility is being socially conscious and making efforts to be a contributing member of your organization and society in general.

DECISION MAKING CLUSTER

> *Judgments and decisions are guided directly by feelings of liking and disliking, with little deliberation or reasoning.*
>
> —DANIEL KAHNEMAN, *THINKING, FAST AND SLOW*

The decision making cluster is about your understanding of how emotions and biases may affect your decision making and help delay your impulses. It includes problem solving, reality testing, and impulse control. This cluster is the most outward representation of your emotional intelligence and can impact the medical risk of professionals. This translates to the following questions:

* Am I able to manage my impulses and reactions in what I say and do?

    ✦   Can I find good solutions when my emotions are aroused?

    ✦   Can I stay objective in spite of the situation?

Impulse control is the ability to stay calm, composed, and patient when there is emotionality in a situation.

Problem solving is the ability to understand how emotions impact decision making and is a systematic way to solve problems.

Reality testing is recognizing when emotions or personal bias can cause you to be less objective. You have limited biases that cloud your decision making.

STRESS MANAGEMENT CLUSTER

> *Should you find yourself in a chronically leaking boat,*
> *energy devoted to changing vessels is likely to be more*
> *productive than energy devoted to patching leaks.*

> —WARREN BUFFETT

The stress management cluster is about how well you can cope with the emotions associated with change, unfamiliar and unpredictable circumstances, while remaining hopeful about the future and resilient in the face of setbacks and obstacles[34]. This cluster includes flexibility, stress tolerance, and optimism, all of which directly influence burnout.

This translates to the following questions:

    ✦   How adaptable am I?

    ✦   How much stress can I handle?

    ✦   What is my attitude when there are difficult circumstances?

Flexibility is effectively adapting your emotions, thoughts, and behaviors to changing circumstances and conditions, and being open to new viewpoints.

Stress tolerance is having effective coping strategies and believing you can manage or influence in dynamic situations in a stable and relaxed manner.

Optimism is remaining hopeful and resilient despite occasional setbacks, while remaining hopeful and confident about the future.

Some Emotional Intelligence Cases
Let's now look at a few examples of burnout and EI in medical practice.

Case 1: Poor Decision Making
Dr. Foster storms into the next operating room after performing a long surgery. He glances briefly at the chart and remembers the patient's name and situation. He then asks for the scalpel to begin the surgery. The operating nurse, Joan Sullivan, meekly asks a clarifying question about the surgery, and Dr. Foster interrupts and barks an order for the next instrument. Joan doesn't inquire again as Dr. Foster performs surgery on the wrong leg.

In which two competencies does Dr. Foster need to dial down this behavior?

1. Problem solving
2. Assertiveness
3. Empathy
4. Independence

In which two competencies does Joan Sullivan need to improve?

1. Self-regard
2. Intrapersonal relations
3. Assertiveness
4. Optimism

CASE 2: DISSATISFIED AND OVERWHELMED

Jim Hansen, Senior Vice President, is in charge of the electronic records initiative. His deliverable is to go live September 1, and he has been working on it nonstop for the last six weeks, until ten o'clock every night and on almost every weekend. He has been unable to get key stakeholders to make his meeting critical to get buy-in from Dr. Penner and his team, who are necessary for the implementation. Dr. Penner had promised that they would have representatives attend, but they missed the last two meetings. Jim now realizes there are not enough hours or resources to meet the deadline. Dr. Penner apologizes, stating he had an emergency come up at the time of the last two meetings. Jim is stressed and wondering if this is the right position for him. He has to report to the oversight committee tomorrow and is anxious and unable to sleep, thinking about what he will say.

In which two competencies does Jim need to improve?

1. Assertiveness
2. Impulse control
3. Self-actualization
4. Expressiveness

In which two competencies does Dr. Penner need to dial up his behavior?

1. Intrapersonal relations
2. Emotional self-awareness
3. Empathy
4. Optimism

CASE 3: POOR PATIENT CARE

Dr. McGorey is rounding on his patient, Mrs. Jones. He slept only three hours last night and has not eaten, and he has an important meeting in twenty minutes. As Mrs. Jones begins to speak, he does not look at her but stares at the chart, trying to focus. He interrupts her and says everything looks good and she does not need to worry. When she asks for clarification, he replies coldly, "Look, I have done this a thousand times. You just have to trust me." He then briskly walks out the door.

In which two competencies does Dr. McGorey need to improve?

1. Independence
2. Empathy
3. Stress Tolerance
4. Self- Regard

In which two competencies does Dr. McGorey need to dial down his behavior?

1. Assertiveness
2. Flexibility
3. Self-regard
4. Intrapersonal relations

CASE 4: STRAINED RELATIONS

Mary Kensey, Chief Nursing Officer, hears about a patient's husband, who is at the hospital to pick up his wife and their newborn, when their car is towed because he parked in a restricted area. Mary is furious, as she is trying to be service oriented and knows this story will be terrible public relations for her birth program. She storms into the office of Ann Miller, the director of Human Resources, demanding the head of security be fired right now as she has had numerous other issues with him. Ann says, "You seem so angry. Can we talk about it so I can understand what happened and help you?" She is able to calm Mary down and talk rationally about the issue, and together they come up with a solution.

In which two competencies does Mary needs to improve?

1. Self-actualization
2. Self-regard
3. Empathy
4. Impulse control

In which two competencies does Ann shine?

1. Optimism
2. Empathy
3. Problem solving
4. Flexibility

EMOTIONAL INTELLIGENCE AND OTHER HEALTHCARE PERSONNEL

As is shown by the case studies above, burnout is prevalent among all healthcare professionals, not just physicians; therefore, EI is necessary for all professionals. EI is a set of skills that is as vital as technical skills are in the medical field, and although most of the research shown has been on physicians, the spectrum of EI and the research conducted on it has targeted all personnel involved in patient care. Nurses, nurse practitioners, physician assistants, and health care executives have also been studied, and the results are no less impressive in terms of the palpable connection, the documented effects, and the potential and measurable outcomes.

In 2008, Codier et al. researched the relationship between EI and nursing staff performance[40]. They found that EI correlates positively with the level of performance of nurses; in simple terms, the higher the EI score, the better the performance across all nursing responsibilities. Further, they found that most nurses score low or below average on total

---

40 Codier E, Kooker BM, Shoultz J. (2008) Measuring the emotional intelligence of clinical staff nurses: an approach for improving the clinical care environment. *Nursing Administration.* 32(1), 8-14.

EI and its sub-scores. By the same analogy used before with physicians, poor EI scores lead to poor performance and outcomes with a direct negative impact on patient satisfaction, health outcomes, and risks.

In 2008, Morrison discovered that for nurses to be able to work effectively and productively in high-stress situations or departments, they need to possess effective and strong conflict-resolution skills[41]. The author found that these skills and abilities, which help nurses not only deal with patients but also with co-workers, managers, physicians, and peers, are strongly and directly related to emotional intelligence. Specifically, through interpersonal and communication skills, EI was shown to be important in conflict resolution and stress management. The author recommends that management needs to incorporate this skill of EI in training and EI awareness.

In 2015, Zhu et al. focused on the organizational engagement of nurses and how involved they are in their workplace[42]. Organizational engagement is of paramount importance and is well documented to have a positive impact on nurses, their performance, their well-being, and their ability to provide quality care. The authors found out that EI and organizational justice are both positive predictors of such an engagement, and they recommended managers enhance and focus on both aspects for better quality of care and staff well-being.

In 2012, Mandle and Schweinle conducted a study on physician assistant students and found that their empathy decreased as they practiced longer[43], following patterns similar to the ones observed in medical students with regard to burnout and empathy. They went on to note that the same issues that affect physicians also influence their assistants due to the commonality of factors, education, and responsibilities.

---

41   Morrison J. (2008) The relationship between emotional intelligence competencies and preferred conflict-handling styles. *Journal of Nursing Management*. 16(8), 974-83.

42   Zhu Y., Liu C., Guo B., Zhao L., Lou F. (2015) The impact of emotional intelligence on work engagement of registered nurses: the mediating role of organisational justice. *Journal of Clinical Nursing*. 24(15-16):2115-24.

43   Mandel, E.D., Schweinle, W.E. (2012) A study of empathy decline in physician assistant students at completion of first didactic year. *The Journal of Physician Assistant Education*. 23(4), 16-24.

Evidently, no healthcare industry worker involved in patient care is spared from the phenomenon of burnout, loss of empathy, and exposure to significant stress. But it is not only healthcare professionals that suffer; perhaps equally important, if not more so, are the executives and managers who are responsible for maintaining departments, hospitals, and healthcare institutions. They too are not spared the rigors and stress, with a major effect on healthcare outcomes.

In 2002, Freshman and Rubino discussed the value of a healthcare leader/executive who possesses high EI skills[44]. In their extensive report, the authors found that leaders who have skills in some of the EI parameters, such as self-awareness, self-regulation and motivation, social awareness, and social skills, were better able to:

1. Confidently manage budgets with better decisions
2. Differentiate between personal and healthcare values that may be different
3. See the importance of their family and their staff's, in conducting and managing meeting times
4. Deal with providers and know when to step away for better outcomes
5. Manage medical billing compliance issues
6. Accept responsibility over other healthcare facilities
7. Be optimistic, embracing diversity and maximizing the potential and abilities of their staff
8. Be more compassionate
9. Be more patient-centered
10. Listen to others and improve employee satisfaction
11. Negotiate healthcare contracts and maximize opportunities for their establishments

---

44 Freshman B., Rubino L. (2002) Emotional Intelligence: A Core Competency for Health Care Administrators. *Health Care Manager.* 20(4), 1–9.

All this has shown that EQ is one explanation for success versus failure of healthcare organizations in terms of delivering patient-centered care. EQ has been shown to positively correlate with:

1. Better physician–patient relationship and interaction
2. Increasing empathy
3. Decreasing burnout
4. Improved communication
5. Improved stress management
6. Improved organizational commitment
7. Improved employee retention
8. Improved staff career satisfaction
9. Improved effective leadership
10. Improved organizational citizenship
11. Improved positive patient outcomes

Emotional Intelligence has been researched extensively in the medical literature. More and more of its science has been recognized as a necessity to the practice of healthcare. Unfortunately, it has also been found to be severely lacking in our training and education. That we know why and how it is needed makes it that much more important to study and properly implement. The data supports its importance. The research calls for its proper use and implementation. Against burnout, it is one of the most important tools we have in detecting the manifestations of this malignancy within us and amongst others.

CHAPTER 8

Wellness, Emotional Intelligence, Balance, and Burnout

• • •

"Life does not get easier or more forgiving, we get stronger and more resilient"

STEVE MARABOLI

IF YOU HAD A SHATTERED leg, resulting in multiple fractures, would you stand on it to work in the operating room, the emergency room, or the clinic? Of course not; the physical pain would be too great. Whether we sustain a minor or major injury, our body tells us something is wrong in a variety of ways, one of which is pain.

Now, what if you had a crushed psyche? What if you were burned out with a fractured brain? Since it would be out of the question to work while bearing weight on a fractured lower extremity, why is it conceivable—and dare we say, expected—to work with a broken mind?

Several factors have led physicians to work while they are burned out, some of which we have discussed. Another major factor we need to look at is awareness. How many physicians are aware that they are burned out?

What would happen if you continued to work on shattered lower extremity? How much pain could you take before you passed out, collapsed, or start taking drugs to numb the pain? How much would you be able to endure before thinking of ending your career—or, even worse, your life? Physical pain is easy to identify and relate to; emotional pain is not so simple. Let's now examine why we not only lack awareness of our emotional pain when burned out, but also why we are actually trained to ignore it!

Think about your medical school and residency training. Whether you are there now, have just graduated, or have been practicing for years, two of the behaviors that are stressed are suppression of emotion and disengagement from the effect of what we do on our emotional well-being. We regard human beings as "cases," thereby emphasizing the need to emotionally distance ourselves from patients while trying to treat them with empathy. Further, we are required to hide our own emotions—to bury them somewhere and not identify with them. This has been a mainstay of training.

Fortunately, this is now changing, with more and more residencies and schools encouraging their students and staff to talk about their feelings, express themselves, and relate. Still, for most people, showing emotions and discussing them is frowned upon due to the perception of weakness and the stigma of not being strong enough or competent enough to be a physician. When did being a physician require us to be robot like in our approach?

Amid all the training on connecting with patients, the stress is that we must not connect with our own emotions, suppressing them instead. With time, that creates a tremendous deficiency in us: our inability to read our own emotional pain.

We previously said that whether pain is emotional, psychosocial, or physical, the brain perceives it as pain. With physical pain, we recognize it immediately as it is a survival signal that must be heeded, but not so with emotional pain. Just ask those suffering from emotional problems about how they are treated by their family and friends and the medical community. When we see someone in a wheelchair, we open the door for them and try to help, but when see someone who is in emotional pain, the reaction is often judgment and condescension.

So here we are, in a profession that stresses suppression of emotions but relies on emotional connection. Our awareness of our emotional state is greatly lacking. With that in mind, let's look at what it means to be more aware and how we can do that.

AWARENESS OF BURNOUT

If you have ever flown a plane, you know that the instruments in the cockpit are what provide you with direction, altitude, and everything else you need to know how to fly, even in total darkness. These instruments give you optics. Likewise, physical pain gives you optics about injury to the body, and emotional intelligence gives you optics about injury to the mind.

The cornerstone of emotional intelligence is to know yourself—or the self-perception realm, of which emotional self-awareness is a part. Once you identify your EQ profile, you can be trained to improve your deficiencies. One of the beauties of EQ, as mentioned earlier, is that unlike IQ, it is a modifiable.

While it is not within the scope of this book to talk about the training techniques involved in enhancing our emotional intelligence, we will say that when we improve our optics, we are able to recognize our emotional pain long before it has deleterious effects on us. Years of training and philosophies of medicine can be reversed and overcome using certain EQ techniques. EQ training allows us to be in touch with who we are and what our body/mind/soul is telling us. And with that, the connection with wellness becomes apparent.

Although recovery from burnout is possible, prevention is a better strategy. As Dr. Shanafelt has mentioned in numerous publications, "Physicians who actively nurture and protect their personal and professional well-being on all levels—physical, emotional, psychological, and spiritual—are more likely to prevent burnout or at least mitigate its consequences. The promotion of personal wellness needs to occur throughout the professional life cycle of physicians, from medical school through retirement"[45]

---

45 Balch C.M., Freischlag J.A., Shanafelt T.D. (2009) Stress and burnout among surgeons: understanding and managing the syndrome and avoiding the adverse consequences. *Archives of Surgery*. 144(4):371-6. doi: 10.1001/archsurg.2008.575.

According to Frank Herbert, "There is no secret to balance. You just have to feel the waves." While he was referring to a surfer trying to conquer a giant wave, his message is truly universal. The key words here are *balance* and *feeling*. Life is about achieving balance. And with that said, let's introduce the concept of balance.

BALANCE

If we were to look up quotes or philosophies about happiness and balance, we would come across so many that address finding the right relationship between career and personal life. Many quotes stress finding meaning in life, not being consumed by our career, and enjoying the blessings we have. But balance is easier said than achieved. Just ask the thousands of physicians practicing medicine. How many, including yourself, will answer that their professional life is balanced with their psychosocial and physical life? They can probably be counted on one hand. And they most likely won't include you! It is no secret that we really do not know how to balance our lives. If we did, we would be a much happier group of professionals who are not so burned out.

Why is balance so important? One word: Wellness.

WELLNESS

The concept of total wellness recognizes that our every thought, word and behavior affects our greater health and wellbeing. And we, in turn, are affected not only emotionally but also physically and spiritually.

—GREG ANDERSON

Whatever our definition of wellness, it is a state of emotional, physical, social, and spiritual existence. Wellness is the sum of all its parts. Some readers may be familiar with the wellness wheel. (The six parts of the wellness wheel are physical, emotional, spiritual, occupational, cognitive/

intellectual, and social) And while it could be considered foolish to try to accomplish wellness in all its facets and parts, it may be more foolish not to!

As physicians, we are at the forefront of trying to help people be well, doing this through prevention and treatment. We diagnose problems, help prevent problems, and treat problems. We also stress to our patients that fighting a disease and being well involves more than just taking medications; it is a way of life. Living healthy is our medical definition of wellness. We focus on healthy lifestyles and healthy interventions. But the reality of wellness is that it encompasses so many facets of who we are, and in the medical profession, our emotional and psychosocial wellness parts are atrociously taken care of.

If emotional intelligence provides us with the optics of emotional pain, emotional and physical wellness help us heal and prevent further injury. They fortify and train us, making us stronger and helping us develop resilience and awareness. An integral part of emotional intelligence is well-being, under which the stress management realm exists. But whereas EQ training helps in our well-being, it may not be enough to help with our overall wellness. And wellness, as we can all attest, is not one of our strong suits. In fact, we make the worst patients! For we, as physicians and healthcare workers, truly do not know how to care for ourselves.

Wellness needs effort. It takes time and commitment. If we can afford so much time and effort to achieve a successful career, why not afford the same time and effort for the other facets of wellness? Some may answer that existence is incompatible with being a physician—and they may be right given everything we have to do to get our job done.

But while our profession demands so much from us on all levels, satisfying the wellness wheel does not. There are exercises, rituals, prayers, and mindsets that one can train in, and they require little time, when compared to the professional commitment we have, but yield tremendous results. Exercising for ten to fifteen minutes a day, eating healthy foods, using prayers, meditation, and mindfulness techniques, and engaging in family time are all extremely rewarding. Wellness is necessary to maintain a great life-and-work balance, and that balance is easily tipped toward work and burnout if we don't take care. Looking at the slide below, perhaps it now makes more sense.

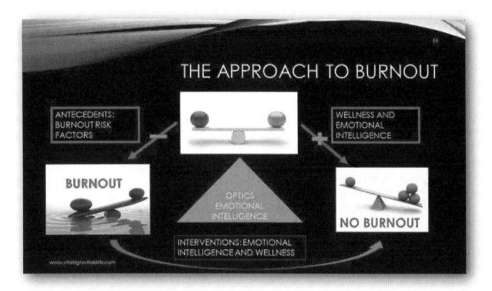

As long we are balanced, we have self-control and our neocortex is in command of our decisions. If the antecedent factors that lead to burnout overwhelm our life, then the balance is tipped to the left and we end up burned out with all its negative consequences. If wellness and emotional intelligence abilities fortify our life, then the balance is tipped to the right and we end up not burned out and leading an even better life. The ability to detect which side dictates our life is described through the optics of emotional intelligence, and once this is determined, we can swing the pendulum from burnout to no burnout by mastering wellness and emotional intelligence.

To summarize, the more work and less wellness, the more the burnout. Maintaining balance is key for wellness, and maintaining wellness is key for a balanced existence. What makes us aware of our burnout is our ability to identify our emotional pain, as seen through our optics instruments (our EQ). Maintaining our EQ and balance requires a solid investment in wellness and EQ training and maintenance. By being well, and by having a high EQ, we are able to balance our life and work, identify burnout, minimize it, combat it, and, perhaps even more importantly, be happy and fulfilled.

In the next chapter, we will put this in the context of our six concepts: burnout, pendulum, emotional intelligence, optics, balance, and wellness.

CHAPTER 9

Wellness/Balance – A Unique Vaccine and Resiliency Equation

• • •

"Balance is not something you find. It is something you create."

JANA KINGSFORD

JUST LIKE WITH INFECTIOUS DISEASES and certain malignancies, vaccines are created to prepare the human body and help its immune system fight. The premise is simple: Introduce the body to part of the disease or causative agent, and allow it to develop the necessary capabilities to fight if it ever encounters i. With wellness, the concept of "immunizing" the body against burnout follows a slightly different pathway; however, the result is making the body strong and resistant to the deleterious effects of burnout.

Resiliency can be defined as the ability to bounce back from difficult times or obstacles in a healthy way. A well-conditioned athlete recovers from injury quickly. A well-prepared student anticipates academic needs better. A well-trained professional is more likely to succeed. And only one aspect of our life is able to make us well conditioned, well prepared, and well trained for burnout: wellness.

This chapter will review some of the literature that discusses the profound effects of wellness and a good work–life balance on preventing and dealing with burnout.

Like any affliction, we do our best to protect against burnout and ensure we are thoroughly prepared so we have the best possible outcome once we encounter it. The past eight chapters have focused on the ways and reasons burnout affects us. Now we are going to look at some of the personal factors that make us susceptible to burnout. We know that female gender, not having a supportive partner, having a type A personality, younger age, being a junior physician, and having traits of compulsiveness and extraversion will predispose us to burnout. Further, having distorted cognitive thought processes such as perfectionism, all-or-none thinking, and unrealistic expectations have also been linked to stress and burnout[46]. These are some of the main reasons why cognitive behavioral therapy works for certain people with burnout. It changes their ways of thinking and the behaviors that follow.

Given all of the above, it seems logical that whatever we can do to build resiliency and better prepare ourselves for the negative effects of burnout will bolster our coping mechanisms as well as our abilities to maintain them. So let's look at a comprehensive definition of wellness and why it is so important to achieve it.

---

46 Orsekovich M., Anderson J. (2013) Physician personalities and burnout. *Bulletin of the American College of Surgeons.* 98(6):40-2.

Wellness

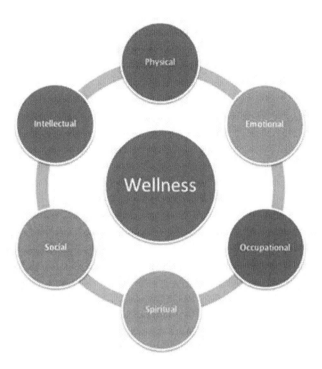

Wellness involves the six realms shown in the diagram. If we take a moment to look at each realm and imagine ourselves being "well" in it, we can understand the effects of each on us as human beings and as physicians. We have already discussed distorted emotions and negative emotional states, and have highlighted the fact that burnout is genotypically an emotionally malignant disease. Now let's explore what the other realms contribute.

Physical Fitness

> *A feeble body weakens the mind."*
>
> —Jean-Jacques Rousseau

Being physically well is not a strange concept to physicians; we preach it all the time. Physically fit people fare better in fighting disease and recovering from a procedure, and are less prone to infections and diseases. Perhaps even more important, a physically fit body creates a much better internal environment for the mind to work; physical fitness leads to mind and cognitive fitness.

OCCUPATIONAL/FINANCIAL FITNESS

As we discuss occupational fitness, you will see how everything is intertwined. If all is "well," then we are well. If things are out of sorts, one realm will impact the others. If we were to define occupational wellness as being happy and satisfied in our work and our profession, then we are in effect dismissing burnout to start with. However, burnout is more complex than just dissatisfaction with our work (although it is affected tremendously by it).

In the grand scheme of burnout, some of the aspects we can discuss here are peer support, time flexibility, decreased demands, and increased autonomy. It behooves us to examine our working environment. Whether we are seeking to sign a contract for a new position, renew an existing one, or simply reevaluate where we are, we must be sure that our working place will not contribute to burnout. A disorganized place, a non-supportive management structure, a non-supportive peer environment, unclear expectations, unrealistic expectations, not enough ancillary support, poor reimbursement or dysfunctional payment systems, difficult call schedules, and suboptimal electronic records and dictation software have all been linked to burnout. Minimizing external factors that will make things worse is a must.

If necessary, we may need to seek a better role in our profession or a better organization and/or position that suits our personalities, our life demands, and our professional expectations.

SPIRITUAL FITNESS

Research has shown that people who practice some type of faith are less prone to burnout and maladaptive and disruptive behaviors, and are in general much more fulfilled. The reasons behind this affect not only burnout, but also people's lives in general. Being fulfilled spiritually translates to increased resilience, increased emotional support from family and community, a more grounded approach to life, and development of a belief system that keeps us connected with ourselves and others. Spiritual well-being also reduces emotional exhaustion and depersonalization. By practicing humility, spirituality, and internal fluidity and connectedness, as well as building a strong relationship with relatives and friends, we can not only decrease burnout but also protect against it.

SOCIAL FITNESS

According to several surveys, the latest from Medscape, physicians' favorite pastimes include spending time with family, traveling, exercising, reading, and attending cultural events. On a professional side, the more a physician has social support networks, the less the burnout. Social connection is not only encouraged, it is recommended, although this trend is now only starting to emerge among physicians.

We go through our training, which stresses certain qualities such as individual accolades and achievements, being up to the tasks expected, and going above and beyond without showing signs of weakness or need. Our culture is as demanding and sometimes unforgiving as it could be, with more of an alpha-male (or alpha-female) mentality and less of a herd existence.

This puts a lot of stress on us, and we are not taught how to foster nurturing professional relationships. In general, studies have shown that the more physicians are connected to their families, friends, and, social circle, the more resilient they are. Further, programs that encourage leisure time and social gatherings among residents, students, and peers have resulted in better attitudes, less burnout, and increased coping abilities.

INTELLECTUAL FITNESS

This book has focused on our intellectual fitness and ensuring that our cognitive abilities are not eroded by our emotional burdens. The cycle comes full circle when we realize that intellectual fitness and whole-body wellness feed off each other. Putting them in context of our profession as physicians provides a different perspective on things, and we see that we are as strong as our weakest link.

Think about which link is your weakest, and then rank your fitness categories from best to worst. Visualize where you currently are, and, more importantly, where you want (or need) to be.

BALANCE AS A PART OF WELLNESS

In medicine, one of the most direct relationships in diseases is the one between hypertension and complications. The higher the blood pressure, the more the complications. That same relationship exists between work balance and burnout. The worse the work-balance relationship, the greater the propensity for burnout. So, the more the demands on us and the fewer the rewards, the less balanced and more burned out we are. To combat this, review of the literature suggests these steps be taken:

1. Identify where you are.
    This stresses self-analysis and determining your place. By clearly identifying where you are, you also identify what is missing, what is negative, and what is positive.
2. List the positive and negative contributors.
    Knowing where you are in the balance is one thing. Knowing how each aspect of your life contributes is another. For example,

spending time with family is a great positive asset. But what is it in particular that maximizes your time with them and gives you the greatest pleasure? Also identify the (negative) contributors to imbalance. As you set your priorities, the most important factors will have to be tackled first. Think about doing chart documentation at work versus at home. Although both are related to work, each carries a different negative "coefficient of importance." While we might prefer to be at home, working while there often leads to increased stress and resentment by you, your spouse, and your children, as you are home but not available to them.

3. Define your true goals and your wants and needs.
   Make a list of your goals, wants, and needs (it is important to achieve not only our needs but also our wants). Making a list and prioritizing will give you an advantage moving forward, primarily due to time constraints.

4. Manage your time wisely.
   Of all the things that time management depends on, other than priorities, being realistic is crucial. Having a good understanding of who you are, what you have, and where you want to go and what it would take, as well as what you need to get there, gives you the best possible chance at balancing your work and life. We all know we cannot and will not have everything we desire and need. So, assigning "coefficient factors" to our needs and prioritizing them, while keeping ourselves grounded in realistic expectations and goals, gives us the best possible chance of balance. In an article published by Gordon and Borkan in 2014[47], the authors recommend four steps for effective time management among physicians:
   * Setting short-term and long-term goals
   * Setting priorities between different responsibilities
   * Planning and organizing activities
   * Minimizing "time wasters"

---

47   Gordon C.E., Borkan S.C. (2014) Recapturing time: a practical approach to time management for physicians. *Postgraduate Medical Journal.* 90(1063), 267-72.

5. Always assess and adjust.

   After you have carefully revised your goals, prioritized your needs and wants, and come up with the best possible time-management formula, the next step is to live out your plans. However, like most best-laid plans, they may not work. Along your road to wellness and balance, develop a habit of pit stops to allow yourself to assess and adjust. See where you are, what you have achieved, and what needs to be tweaked or changed completely. Analyze your failures, celebrate and replicate your successes, and keep on the path. Often, we are forced to not modify our approaches, but completely change the path. And that is fine too. For as long we do not lose sight of our primary objectives—to live well, reduce burnout, and excel at our profession—we can be flexible to analyze, accommodate, and react.

RESILIENCE AS A PART OF WELLNESS

In 2013, an article by Epstein and Krasner looked at resiliency among physicians[48]. After defining resiliency as the ability to bounce back from challenges while learning from them and becoming stronger, they cited resilience factors, which include practicing mindfulness, monitoring one's self, setting limits, and possessing attitudes that encourage healthy and constructive approaches to challenges at work rather than running away from them. While we wait for institutions and academies and programs to install a community-fostering and resilience-building program, it remains up to us as individuals to learn how to develop these skills.

The American Psychological Association (APA) offers these 10 ways to build resilience quoted directly from the source:

1. **Make connections.** "Accepting help and support from those who care about you and will listen to you strengthens resilience."

---

48 Epstein RM, Krasner MS. (2013) *Physician Resilience: what it means, why it matters, and how to promote it.* Academic Medicine. 88(3), 301-3.

2. **Avoid seeing crises as insurmountable problems.** "Try looking beyond the present to how future circumstances may be a little better."

3. **Accept that change is a part of living.** "Accepting circumstances that cannot be changed can help you focus on circumstances that you can alter."

4. **Move toward your goals.** "Do something regularly—even if it seems like a small accomplishment—that enables you to move toward your goals."

5. **Take decisive actions.** "Rather than detaching completely from problems and stresses and wishing they would just go away, act on adverse situations as much as you can."

6. **Look for opportunities for self-discovery.** "People often learn something about themselves and may find that they have grown in some respect as a result of their struggle with loss."

7. **Nurture a positive view of yourself.** "Developing confidence in your ability to solve problems and trusting your instincts helps build resilience."

8. **Keep things in perspective.** "Even when facing very painful events, try to consider the stressful situation in a broader context and keep a long-term perspective."

9. **Maintain a hopeful outlook.** "Try visualizing what you want, rather than worrying about what you fear."

10. **Take care of yourself.** "Pay attention to your own needs and feelings. Engage in activities that you enjoy and find relaxing."

CHAPTER 10

Tools for Fighting Burnout

• • •

"In a battle all you need to make you fight is a little hot blood and
the knowledge that it's more dangerous to lose than to win."

GEORGE BERNARD SHAW

IN GOING THROUGH THE BURNOUT transformation of a physician, we have discussed the why and the what as well as the how and the when, touching on the internal and external factors. Fighting burnout starts within, and the first step is awareness. Acceptance and acknowledgement can only happen within each of us, but the hope is that we have provided the necessary optics to do so. In theory, the action is to improve EQ and practice self-care. This chapter deals with some of the approaches to assist with that.

CONSCIOUS ATTENTIONAL DEPLOYMENT AND INFLUENCE

In a major review of 128 studies on positive interventions looking at emotional regulation strategies[49], Quoidbach, Mikolajczak, and Gross found that attentional deployment before, during, and after a positive emotional

---

49 Quoidbach, Mikolajczak and Gross (2015) Positive Interventions: An Emotion Regulation Review. *Psychological Bulletin*, American Psychological Association.

event received strong empirical support and were the center of many positive interventions. They defined attentional deployment by stating that "the way we direct our attention within a situation can powerfully influence our emotional experience." Where we focus our attention greatly influences our mood, happiness, and satisfaction.

Other evidence of the power of mastering the moment comes from Robert Cialdini, Ph.D., an expert on influence theory and author of *Influence: The Psychology of Persuasion*. He has added to the influence theory with *Pre-Suasion: A Revolutionary Way to Influence and Persuade*, written about the concept of "pre-suasion," or the priming before the influence[50]. He states, "Consequential effects of shift in focus, in that moment we grant the focal factor importance, assign it causal status and undertake actions associated with it." He also states, "Mental activity fires when readied. Once a concept receives attention, closely associated secondary concepts become more accessible in consciousness, which generally improves the chance that we will attend and respond to the linked concept. The newly enhanced standing in consciousness elevates their capacity to color our perceptions, orient our thinking, affect our motivations and thereby change our relevant behavior."

ATTENTION MANAGEMENT

The goal is to be more in charge of your focus and attention, sometimes called "attention management." Brain neuroscientists have shown that the way to change our brain is with attention and focus. Most of the time we are operating on autopilot, so our focus is episodic and undisciplined. Having emotional intelligence means being in charge of reactions and, in the moment, having more choices, making better judgments and decisions, and communicating more effectively. Below are key strategies to give more clarity to insight and empathy.

---

50 Cialdini, R. (2016) *Pre-Suasion: A Revolutionary Way to Influence and Persuade*. New York: Simon and Shuster.

SELF-PERCEPTION

Emotional self-awareness is knowing when and why an emotion will be triggered and knowing how to use that emotion to your benefit; it is the starting point for improving your emotional intelligence. We use the dictum that awareness equals responsibility, meaning if you are aware, you can take more responsibility for your choices and therefore your results. Responsibility can be broken down to the "ability to respond." So, the more awareness you have the more choices and responses are available to you in the moment; more of your IQ points are available for your decision making.

Glenn Rifkin, via the Korn Ferry Institute, analyzed almost 7000 self-assessments from professionals at 486 publicly traded companies based on rate of return and frequency of blind spots[51]. They found:

* Poor performing companies' employees had 20 percent more blind spots than financially strong companies.
* Poor performing companies were 79 percent more likely to have low overall self-awareness.
* People with fewer blind spots had improved performance and greater satisfaction.

So, how do you raise your emotional self-awareness? One helpful tool comes from the research of Dr. Richard Davidson, who looked at different emotional styles. Knowing which style you are can help you accept it and modify it if you need to[52].

Look at the styles below decide which you are. It is also helpful, for the empathy side of the equation, to decide where those you work closely with fall.

1. Start-up (fast, medium, or slow)
   When something goes awry, how fast or slow is your reaction? Do you immediately react and start releasing stress hormones (fast), or are you not easily aroused by the unexpected (slow)?

---

51 https://www.kornferry.com/institute/filling-your-blind-spots
52 Davidson and Begley (2012): *Emotional Life of Your Brain.* New York: Penguin Group.

2. Intensity (high, medium, low)
    What is the strength of your reaction? Do you blow your top (high), or do you have a mild and tempered reaction (low)?
3. Duration (long, medium, short)
    Once you react, how long does it stay with you? Do you get over it quickly (short), or do you let a perceived rejection fester (long)?

SELF-EXPRESSION

Emotional expressiveness can be defined as the action part of the emotional experience[34]. The brain is always making associations, so in speaking, can you be deliberate about what you want to say and what associations you are linking?

Andrew Newberg, M.D. and Mark Robert Waldman say words can literally change your brain[53]: "A single word has the power to influence the expression of genes that regulate physical and emotional stress." If you are on autopilot, you may blurt out something that puts the person on the defensive. Their body then releases cortisol and other stress neurochemicals that lead to distrust. The authors recommend that you express appreciations, speak warmly, speak slowly, and speak briefly (thirty-second chunks are about as much information as we can hold in short-term memory). Then pause and see what questions or responses the other person has before you go on.

We tell our clients to focus on having three positive comments for every negative one. The negative is usually so powerful that it takes three positive statements to counteract it. Use this as a metric for yourself, to be more conscious of the amount of positive comments you are giving your co-workers and family members.

Another tool that can help increase your ration is the POWRR tool. Here you turn any success into a process so it can be repeated. It stands for **P**oint **O**ut **W**hat was **R**ight and you want **R**epeated. This focus of

---

53 Newberg A. and Waldman, M.R. (2012). *Words Can Change Your Brain*. New York: Penguin Group.

attention on what was right gives more weight to what is positive and allows for the action to be repeated. Using the word *because* compels you to come up with specific actions or steps for the individuals to repeat. For example: "Many thanks for getting the report down so fast, *because* now we will have time to think of all the people to distribute it to.

"It helped that you came to me early to clarify the scope as many people feel I may be too busy to come see. I like that you collaborated with so many people on it and that worked last one night last week. Your presentation of the material was flawless and my boss took note of it also."

Do you see how there is information in this example for what one should do again to be successful? Cialdini highlights this by writing, "what is more accessible in the mind becomes more probable in action."[50]

INTERPERSONAL

Interpersonal relationships describe developing and maintaining mutually satisfying relationships that you have built up or are currently building up, including a useful network of colleagues and professionals. In your relationships, are you authentic? Do you know people on a personal level and feel at ease with people and look forward to engaging in social interactions?[34]

Empathy is recognizing, understanding, and appreciating how other people feel. It involves being able to articulate your understanding of another's perspective and behaving in a way that respects others' feelings.[34] Empathy builds trust and strong relationships because people feel that you see them and know them. Author Stephen Covey has said that listening is to the relationship as breathing is to the body.[54]

So how do you increase your interpersonal relations and empathy?

The "Empathy Audit" is a pre-suasion strategy to activate your mental activity about what may be happening with others. This pre-action will

---

54 Covey S. (2013) *The 7 Habits of Highly Effective People: Powerful lessons in personal change.* Simon & Schuster; Anniversary edition.

prime you for having more intelligence about what to ask, say, or recommend. To do this, ask yourself the questions below when you are having a conversation. The Empathy Audit questions are prefrontal cortex strategic questions that forces you to think and assess what might be going on for another. Ask the questions and wait 3-5 seconds and see what answers emerge for you. You can also ask the person these questions to get their responses to validate your ideas or discover what is happening for them.

* What are they thinking?
* What are they feeling?
* What do they want to happen now?
* How may they (or I) be getting in their (or my) way?
* What do I need to do, or what do they need to do, now that I have this information?

Decision making is finding solutions to challenges and being objective in reviewing information.[34] Lack of impulse control can be one of the fastest ways to derail by making impulsive bad decisions.

Impulse control involves understanding the appropriate times and ways to act on emotions and impulses, and the importance of thinking before acting.[34]

The "Emotional Audit" is an excellent tool to understand yourself and manage your impulses, bringing clarity to the moment. Just like the Empathy Audit can help you understand others, the Emotional Audit helps you understand yourself.

Use the Emotional Audit, when you are triggered by something, to unearth your patterns of behavior. These five questions are prefrontal cortex questions that bring to the forefront what is going on for you. The questions bring blood and oxygen to this area.

It can be used for self-awareness and self-control.

The goal is to take a deep breath and exhale, then ask the following questions, pausing for an answer to rise in your consciousness: The more you do it you are looking for patterns in questions 1, 2 and 4.

- What am I thinking?
- What am I feeling?
- What do I want to happen now?
- How am I getting in my own way?
- What do I need to do differently now?

Triggers are the things people do that get you upset, irritated, or short-tempered. Look at the list below and identify your key triggers (or add yours to this list):

- Being late
- Interrupting you
- Making mistakes
- Talking too much
- Being incompetent
- Being inconsiderate or rude
- Not listening
- Being arrogant and thinking they are always right
- Not working hard and taking easy way out

Now let's look at a case study to demonstrate triggers and the Emotional Audit:

John was known as a "hot head" and had been working on managing his impulse control. At a sales conference, he was giving a presentation as the department head and lost it with his team members, who started looking at e-mails on their computers during his talk. He had asked them to close their computers earlier, and it was the last straw when they opened them again. In the middle of his speech, he yelled at them to close the computers. Afterward, all that anyone remembered was that John lost it again. What happened?

His trigger was that he thought they were being rude, inconsiderate, and disrespectful. Deconstructing this lost moment, John used the Emotional Audit to learn what happened:

1. What was I thinking? *I already told them to close the computer. What are they doing? How rude.*
2. What was I feeling? *Disrespected, angry, and embarrassed.*
3. What did I want? *For them to close the computers and pay attention.*
4. How did I get in my way? *By exploding at them in front of my audience.*
5. What did I need to differently? *Breathe, think, and quietly ask them to close the computer with a slight hand movement.*

John's leadership and credibility took a big hit in this five-second outburst, leading to the opposite of "mastering the moment." Knowing his triggers and having a different response in the moment could have kept this derailing experience from happening.

How does this translate into the medical field? What could trigger such events in different scenarios? A surgeon in the operating room? An emergency room physician in a code blue? An obstetrician trying to deliver a baby? A hospitalist rounding?

Each one of us has his or her own story. If you stop for a moment, can you recall a similar situation? Do you remember when you were "hijacked", had an emotional outburst and the consequences of what happened? Did this happen today, yesterday, a week, a month or a year ago? Can you ask yourself similar questions and come up with answers?

Stress Tolerance is the ability to cope with and respond effectively to stress and mounting pressure, maintaining a level of work performance even under mounting pressure or competition[34]. Many people see stress as bad, and even saying, "I am so stressed," will release cortisol and other neurochemicals. Then there are people who don't see stress as bad, but as part of their performance preparation. Below are ways you can increase stress tolerance:

1. Reframe the stress by telling yourself:
   - "This is a challenge, not a threat."
   - "This is a very meaningful endeavor, and I want to do well at it."
   - "This stress feeling is preparing me to do my best."
   - "My resources are being channeled to help me focus."

In a study from Kelly McGonigal's book *The Upside of Stress*, she reports putting people in the stressful situation of giving a speech to critical judges[55]. Some people saw a three-minute video on how stress is bad. Other people saw three-minute video citing the virtues of stress. The people who saw the "stress is good" video had decreased cortisol and increased HCA, a growth hormone tested with a saliva wipe. The group watching the "stress is bad" video had the opposite results, with increased cortisol and decreased HCA. This change in their biology occurred with a three-minute reframe of stress. Considering this, what kind of mental activity and physiological reaction are you causing with your views on stress?

2. Set up a worry-free zone.
   EQ-i 2.0 action strategies for stress tolerance include:
   * Declare a worry-free zone somewhere in your workplace.
   * Move away from your desk/work area and spend five minutes in a different location (e.g., cafeteria, outside) where the only rule is: No thinking about the thing that is causing you stress.
   * Allow your mind to cool down and become clear again. Only then are you in the best position to leverage your emotions and respond appropriately to the stress[34].

WELLNESS TOOLS

Wellness, or self-care, is self-explanatory. There are many definitions. The most obvious one is that self-care incorporates personal health (along all the wellness wheel dimensions) coupled with a personal/professional balance. The Personal Wellness Foundation tool developed by Well Coaches is an excellent guide for staying well[56]. It states:

---

55 McGonical K. (2015) *The upside of stress, why stress is good for you, and how to get good at it*. Penguin Random House: New York.

56 http://www.wellcoach.com/memberships/images/Chapter-12.pdf

- Self-Care: To support your *best energy*, routinely practice regular self-care.
- Environment: Without any tolerations, design environments that support your *best self.*
- Relationships: Identify the best relationships that support your *best intentions* by connecting with others and yourself.
- Thoughts: To support your *best presence*, adopt values, self-talk, integrity, and attitudes that allow you to do so.
- Time: To support your *highest priorities*, manage your energy over time and spend time wisely.
- Finances: Build reserves and handle money in a way that allow you to give and receive freely.

Here is what we know about wellness among physicians thus far:

- There is an explicit and expected need to develop resident and physician wellness by the ACGME and Clinical Learning Environment Review systems.
- Most research on physician mental/emotional/psychological wellness, which is few and far in between, focuses on cognitive behavioral therapy and mindfulness techniques.
- Clear and effective curricula to enhance and practice wellness are almost nonexistent and are experimental at times.
- Enhancing wellness and promoting it requires the collaboration of physicians and organizations; it is a joint effort.
- Physician wellness has decreased, and burnout symptoms have increased over the past two decades.

Some of the things that most impact physician wellness in a negative way include:

- Workload
- Work efficiency
- Control/flexibility

- Values alignment
- Meaning in work
- Work–life balance

Research has shown that targeting the following would help improve self-care and reduce burnout:

- Stress-reduction training
- Relaxation techniques
- Time management
- Assertiveness training
- Meditation
- Work–life balance measures (hobbies, family, and social activities)
- Self-care measures (physical activity, rest, healthy eating habits)

These all feed into our positive psyche, increase and improve our resilience and coping abilities, and make us better able to handle burnout and stress. While stress is not the same as burnout, stress does contribute to burnout. Stress reduction, assertiveness, relaxation techniques, time management, and meditation are all tied up together. Let's now look at some wellness activities.

Wellness Activity #1

1. On a piece of paper, write down five inexpensive self-care activities (sponge bath, watching TV, reading a book, etc.).
2. Write down five activities that require planning and money (vacation, weekend getaway, going fishing, etc.).
3. Decide how you can fit at least one activity per week into your schedule. The wellness activity time is sacred. Nothing will interrupt you while performing surgery, dealing with a code, or delivering a baby, and this activity requires that commitment. Once

you fit it into your schedule, do it every week. The ideal situation is to have one inexpensive activity and one planned activity per week.

WELLNESS ACTIVITY #2:

1. On a piece of paper, use a scale of 0 to 10 (0 being the least and 10 being the most) to write down your personal wellness score for each realm using the wheel below.
2. Identify one activity that you can do to improve your score along each realm.
3. Set a plan of action to achieve that activity.
4. Complete the activity.

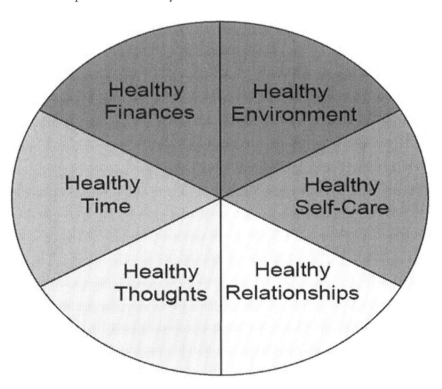

The goal is for the wheel to be smooth and not rough-edged. A 10 puts you on the circumference of the wheel, and a 0 puts you at its center. If your scores range from 4 to 6, for example, then your wheel is going to look jagged and will not turn. Keep adding activities until your wheel is at 10 all around. You will feel and see the difference, as your scores will directly reflect on your wellness and its positive consequences.

WELLNESS ACTIVITY #3

Setting standards and personal boundaries is important for our wellness.

- Personal standards: Standards you hold yourself to.
- Personal boundaries: Boundaries you hold others to.
  - Are made up of imaginary lines that are meant to hold others at a safe distance.
  - Cannot be seen by others if you do not make them known.
  - Are essential to keep unwanted and damaging behavior away from you.
  - Are essential and necessary for self-care.
    - Examples:
      - Others may not yell at me.
      - Others may not speak to me rudely.
      - Others may not enter my office without knocking.
      - Others may not call me at home to discuss office matters.
      - Others may not gossip in my presence.
- Steps to enforce your boundaries:
  - Inform others.
  - Make a request.
  - Give a warning.
  - Follow through with the stated consequence.
  - Let go of the outcome.
    High standards + Clear boundaries = Excellent self-care

1. Write five behaviors/actions that affect you negatively and you wish to block others from doing in your own space.
2. Write five standards that you want to live up to and maintain no matter what.
3. Describe one or two instances when you were forced to sacrifice the boundary of your standard.

WELLNESS ACTIVITY #4

Physicians continue to grow and develop and learn. To develop a professional development plan:

1. Assess your professional skills on a scale of 0 to 10.
2. Set up your intended outcomes (where you want to be in six to twelve months).
3. Develop an action plan to do so—what are you going to do and when? (read, how-skill practice, conferences, CMEs, etc.).
4. Set up a review time and assess.
5. Celebrate your successes, learn from them, and repeat.

WELLNESS ACTIVITY #5

Readiness for change: To help understand your stage of readiness, complete the quiz below.

1. The goal or behavior I want to address first is:
2. My reasons for wanting to change this behavior are:
3. The challenges that I must deal with in changing this behavior are:
4. My strategies for dealing with those challenges are:
5. My goal for next week with respect to this behavior is:
6. My readiness to change this behavior is (indicate yes beside the level that best describes where you are):

a. I won't do it _____
b. I can't do it _____
c. I may do it _____
d. I will do it _____
e. I am doing it _____
f. I am still doing it _____

Practicing self-care and being emotionally intelligent takes effort. As physicians, human beings, partners, parents, supervisors, and leaders, we are obliged by the necessity of life, by our duty to loved ones, by our oath to patients, and by our promise to our students and staff, to care for ourselves first and have the insight and know-how to discover burnout and tackle it. This must be a constant effort that never lets up because our profession never lets up; as long as we are in these roles, wellness and emotional intelligence are demanded, expected, and owed.

Until the powers that be help curtail and positively impact the antecedent factors that lead to burnout, we must remain in control of our own selves. It is within that control that we can face burnout, create the necessary change, and enjoy our life again on a personal and professional level so we can protect and enhance the lives of each other, ourselves, our family and friends, and our patients.

CHAPTER 11

A Patient's Perspective

• • •

"The good physician treats the disease; the great
physician treats the person who has the disease."

William Osler

WITH ALL THE TALK ABOUT physician burnout and its impact on personal and professional lives, let's take a step back and put ourselves in the patient's position. There are many ways to assess how patients receive us as people and as professionals. In fact, this is so important that, as described earlier, an entire medical practice assessment/revenue system is based on it. Hospitals, administrators, and large groups want us to say the right thing and act in a certain way to maintain good Press Ganey or HCAHPS scores. But if we are to follow our code and honor our oath, all these requests are inherently present within the physician interaction with the patient.

Let's perform the following exercise. This is something we ask of our medical students and residents many times, and it is amazing the impact it has. We ask them, especially when rounding on patients, to lie on the stretcher and pretend to be the patient. Just from that perspective, things change. Students and residents suddenly realize a few things.

They feel vulnerable and, because they do not know what is going to happen, are apprehensive. Further, due to their medical knowledge of physicians and the system, they become skeptical and resistant to total submission to healthcare providers. They almost become hostile toward nurses and physicians, relating that to a lack of trust, lack of communication, and fear of the competency (or lack thereof) of the treating nurse and physician. All because they are just pretending to be patients.

We now want to ask you, the reader, to envision yourself as a patient in a clinic, emergency room, or operating room. For this exercise to be effective, you need to fully live the experience in your mind. We have all been a patient at some point in our life, and most of us have once trusted a primary care physician. Some of us see an internist, cardiologist, surgeon, oncologist, or obstetrician. We have all been under the care of someone else.

I remember when I had a small same-day operative procedure and had never met the anesthesiologist before. I kept wondering who he was, how good he was, and what his credentials were. Would I trust him? What if something bad happened? How did I know for sure that he was capable of caring for me? It was tough to fully trust another individual. Now, let me expound on that.

Suppose that anesthesiologist was burned out. Knowing what I know about this ailment, how much trust do you think I would have in him? I would have probably insisted on seeing another physician. Wouldn't you? What if it was your significant other who was going under the knife and you noticed that the physicians were burned out? Would you trust them fully? Knowing what you know now, how would you react? Keep in the back of your mind that you know the science and the procedure, and you can anticipate what will happen.

THE "ME AS A PATIENT" SURVEY

Now try to imagine being a patient and having an unfamiliar physician walk into your room. What would you like to see/feel/hear from this physician? Being fully honest, make a list of all the behaviors you would look for. Once your list is complete, grade yourself as a physician on each behavior, using a scale of 1 to 10, with 10 being a behavior you always exhibit and 1 being a behavior you never exhibit. See how much you fulfill your own requirements. Now score the behaviors while imagining yourself on a burned-out day. Once you do, go back to the role of being a patient and consider how you would feel being treated by you.

The single most important pillar between physician and patient relationship is trust. Trust is earned. Now that you know the behaviors necessary for patients to trust you as their physician, be sure you practice them!

CHAPTER 12

ACEing the Change

• • •

"Before you are a leader, success is all about growing yourself.
When you become a leader, success is all about growing others."

JACK WELCH

IN THIS FINAL CHAPTER, OUR most important question is where do we go from here? With the knowledge we have and the challenges we face, how do we proceed? What are the steps to take during the "Action" phase? Thus far we have spoken about the steps one can take on an individual level. What about the working environment?.

Regardless of whether you work with one partner, a small group, a hospital-based group, or a whole health system, you will need to take efficient and productive action steps. These steps are a summation of what can be found in the literature. They are a reflection and a counter measure to the factors that lead to burnout. Remember that interventions need to happen on an individual, institutional, and group level. Once a decision has been made to intervene, it is imperative that you ACE it:

1. Announce it: Let everyone know that an intervention will happen.
2. Communicate it: Keep everyone informed about what will happen, and give them a road map and goals.

3. Enforce it: Remain steadfast in your approach. Obstacles and challenges await and may be daunting at first. Remember that there are many barriers to break through, and try to get people on board with the approach and program. The good thing is that this "boulder" will roll downhill after the initial effort to move it.

How do you ace it?

Step 1
Identify a champion. Once you realize that burnout it prevalent, something needs to be done about it. Without a champion (a lead person) for that cause, very few things, if any, will be accomplished. Someone will need to adopt this problem and be the lead treating person. That person would run the show and be responsible for the next steps to follow.

Step 2
Assess the damage. Decide which screening tool you will use and screen everyone. Screening should be an annual (or semi-annual) tool, unless there are exceptions, like having an intervention that would necessitate a different time line. Once the prevalence and severity of burnout are identified, further steps can be taken.

Step 3
Get management involved. No matter the structure of your practice, without management invested in combating burnout, the information will remain anecdotal and informative at best. Management must buy in to what needs to happen. Getting them involved can be difficult, but without their support, both financial and managerial, there will be more obstacles

than solutions. While it is beyond the scope of this book to discuss in detail how to get management involved, here are a few points that may help:

- Return on investment: Data shows that it is much more cost effective to retain physicians and working staff than to go through a hiring process. Management knows this firsthand, so show that such interventions increase physician/nurse retention.

- Increased revenue: Getting paid based on physician interaction with the patient (for example, Press Ganey and HCAHPS scores) makes this an easy conversation. The more burned out physicians are, the worse they perform. The better physicians perform and the more empowered they feel, the less burned out they are, which leads to more positive interactions and higher the scores.

- Decreased mistakes: We know that medical errors occur because of the effects of burnout on communication, professionalism, cognitive and physical performances, and patient interaction. Therefore, decreasing burnout decreases mistakes and lawsuits and lowers premiums. It also improves the reputations of hospitals and care providers alike.

- Improved efficiency and decreased length of stay: From a hospital's point of view, nothing decreases revenue more than increased length of a patient's stay. By increasing efficiency and decreasing laxity, by increasing enthusiasm and decreasing complacency, and by improving absenteeism and decreasing presenteeism, revenues improve tremendously.

STEP 4

Develop a culture. According to one of the gurus in management and business, Peter Drucker, "Culture eats strategy for breakfast". One of the key factors to helping burned-out healthcare providers is having a support system and a positive culture. Belonging to a group, feeling protected and supported, and having the freedom, security, and support to discuss and connect with others have all been shown to help combat burnout. That change in culture is easier said than done, but it is becoming more and more the necessary norm. Fear and shame will keep most people from even thinking about this, but once a champion takes charge and creates support channels, organizes group activities, increases the awareness, and discusses the problems, their task becomes that much easier. From experience and data, people will join and become part of that new culture as well as strong advocates for it.

Step 5

Evaluate personal abilities and state of being. Some may see this step as unnecessary, but the logic behind it is that implementing the above changes will be sufficient to create the necessary impact to combat burnout. There is no data or argument to contradict that logic. However, using the same data and logic, the best benefits come from fully evaluating people's abilities and their state of being. The cornerstones of intervention have been emotional intelligence and wellness. One cannot fix what is broken unless one knows the quality and quantity of the break. To do so, outside help is sometimes needed in the form of wellness and executive coaches, support entities, and guiding professionals. There is no greater intervention than the one that targets directed goals, so we recommend that all healthcare workers take an EQ test and have a thorough wellness evaluation.

Step 6

Assess and reassess. To do so, first identify your target goals, then create an action plan with dates, times, and approaches. Further, create a system that assesses your approaches. One CEO asked about such milestones or metrics, and the answer was HCAHPS, Press Ganey, length of stay (LOS), and employee retention. This is usually quite an undertaking, and depending on the size of your group can be quite challenging, so get help from experts in the field, if you need it. Understanding the complexity of burnout, how it permeates, and all the factors involved makes it that much more evident that, at least in the beginning, one needs help. Several approaches have focused on that.

One such program, "Train the Trainer," was adapted by the authors in two separate situations: at an academic center in Texas and with a private hospitalist group in Texas respectively. The results were extremely positive, evident, and sustainable after at least 9 months. Once the system was in place and the approaches, communications, plans, and goals were set, the champion(s) or the program director(s) took over.

STEP 7

Personalize it. Each organization and culture is different; each working environment has its own peculiarities and nuances. Although the scheme is universal, the application is individualized. Knowing what needs to be done is one thing; knowing how to make it work is another. And one cannot optimize any process without taking into consideration the field of application. From assistants, to rules and regulations, to physical space and available funds, to schedules and responsibilities, successful outcomes are highly dependent on the establishment itself. No one is more qualified to individualize the approach as the champion, and as with any leadership role, success depends on how much people will get involved. Involvement is at a much higher rate when people and institutions identify with the process as their own unique approach.

Physician burnout is a contagious malignancy bourn from the demands and reality of the noblest of professions. It eats at the very fabric of medicine (caring for another human being) and destroys both physician and patient alike. Environmental and individual factors play different roles. This disease is upon us with consequences that demand immediate attention. Taking charge of this malignancy, fighting back, and finding solutions starts with creating awareness, acknowledging its existence, and acting. Emotional intelligence and self-care/wellness are two action step modalities that are available, achievable, and proven to be highly effective. It is our moral and ethical duty to take these steps…and fix the fabric.

REFERENCES

• • •

1. Holmboe E.S., Edgar L., Hamstra S. *The Milestones Guidebook.* ACGME publication. 2016.

2. Shanafelt T.D., Hasan O., Dyrbye L.N., Sinsky C., Satele D., Sloan J., West CP. (2015) Changes in Burnout and Satisfaction With Work-Life Balance in Physicians and the General US Working Population Between 2011 and 2014. *Mayo Clinic Proceedings.* 90(12), 1600-13.

3. Medscape lifestyle report 2017: Race and ethnicity, bias and burnout. http://www.medscape.com/features/slideshow/lifestyle/2017

4. Graham J. (2016) Why are doctors plagued by depression and suicide? A crisis comes into focus. https://www.statnews.com/2016/07/21/depression-suicide-physicians/

5. Dyrbye L.N., Thomas M.R., Massie S., Power D.V., Eacker A., Harper W., Durning S., Moutier C., Szyldo D.W., Movotny P.J., Sloan J.A., Shanafelt T.D. (2008) Burnout and Suicial Ideation among Medical Students. *Annals of Internal Medicine.* 149, 334-41.

6. Brauser D. (2015) Impact of burnout: Clinicians speak out. *http://www.medscape.com/viewarticle/839533*

7. Balch C.M., Freischlag J.A., Shanafelt T.D.(2009) Stress and Burnout Among Surgeons: Understanding and Managing the Syndrome and Avoiding the Adverse Consequences. *Archives of Surgery.* 144(4):371-376. doi:10.1001/archsurg.2008.575

8. Williams M., Hevelone N., Alban R.F., Hardy J.P., Oxman D.A., Garcia E., Thorsen C., Frendl G., Rogers S.O. Jr. (2010) Measuring communication in the surgical ICU: better communication equals better care. *Journal of the American College of Surgery.* 210(1):17-22. doi: 10.1016/j.jamcollsurg.2009.09.025. Epub 2009 Oct 28.

9. https://www.cms.gov/medicare/quality-initiatives-patient-assessment-instruments/value-based-programs/macra-mips-and-apms/macra-mips-and-apms.html

10. Stein S.J., Book H.E. (2011) The EQ Edge: Emotional Intelligence and Your Success Paperback. Jossey-Bass. 3rd Edition. ISBN-10: 0470681616

11. Shanafelt T.D., Mungo M., Schmitgen J., Storz K.A., Reeves D., Hayes S.N., Sloan J.A., Swensen S.J., Buskirk S.J. (2016) Longitudinal Study Evaluating the Association Between Physician Burnout and Changes in Professional Work Effort. *Mayo Clinic Proceedings.* 91(4), 422-31.

12. Balch C.M., Shanafelt T. (2011) Combating stress and burnout in surgical practice: a review. *Thoracic Surgery Clinics,* 21(3), 417-30.

13. Goleman D. (2002). Primal Leadership. Harvard Business Press 2002.

14. Cherry, M.G., Fletcher, I., O'Sullivan, H., Dornan, T. (2014) Emotional intelligence in medical education: a critical review. *Medical Education.* 48(5), 468-78.

15. Satterfield, J., Swenson, S., Rabow, M. (2009) Emotional Intelligence in Internal Medicine Residents: Educational Implications for Clinical Performance and Burnout. *Annals of Behavioral Science and Medical Education.* 14(2), 65-68.

16. Ciarrochi JV, Chan AYC, Caputi P. (2000) A critical evaluation of the emotional intelligence construct. *Personality and Individual Differences.* 28:539–561.

17. Taylor, C., Farver, C., Stoller, J.K. (2011) Perspective: Can emotional intelligence training serve as an alternative approach to teaching professionalism to residents? *Academic Medicine.* 86(12), 1551-4.

18. Weng H.C., Hung C.M., Liu Y.T., Cheng Y.J., Chang C.C., Huang C.K. (2011) Associations between emotional intelligence and doctor burnout, job satisfaction and patient satisfaction. *Medical Education.* 45, 835-42.

19. Stoller J.K., Taylor C.A., Farver C.F.(2013) Emotional intelligence competencies provide a developmental curriculum for medical training. *Medical Teacher.* 35(3), 243-7.

20. Mintz L.J., Stoller J.K. (2014) A systematic review of physician leadership and emotional intelligence. *Journal of Graduate Medical Education.* 6(1), 21-31.

21. Constantine M.G., Gainor K.A. (2001) Emotional intelligence and empathy: Their relation to multicultural counseling knowledge and awareness. *Professional School of Counseling.* 5:131–137.

22. Schutte N.S., Schuettpelz E., Malouff J.M. (2001) Emotional intelligence and task performance. *Imagination, Cognition, and Personality.* 20:347–354.

23. McManus IC, Smithers E, Partridge P, Keeling A, Fleming PR. (2003) A levels and intelligence as predictors of medical careers in UK doctors: 20 year prospective study. *British Medical Journal.* 327:139–142.

24. Cherry, M.G., Fletcher, I., O'Sullivan, H., Dornan, T. (2014) Emotional intelligence in medical education: a critical review. *Medical Education.* 48(5), 468-78.

25. Taylor, C., Farver, C., Stoller, J.K. (2011) Perspective: Can emotional intelligence training serve as an alternative approach to teaching professionalism to residents? *Academic Medicine.* 86(12), 1551-4.

26. Schneider S., Kingslover K., Rosdahl J. (2014) Physician coaching to enhance well-being: a qualitative analysis of a pilot intervention. *Explore.* 10(6):372-9.

27. Webb A.R., Young R.A., Baumer J.G. (2010) Emotional Intelligence and the ACGME competencies. *Journal of Graduate Medical Education.* 508-12.

28. Arora S., Ashrafian H., Davis R., Athansiou T., Darzi A., Sevdalis N. (2010) Emotional intelligence in medicine: a systematic review through the context of the ACGME competencies. Medical Education. 44, 749-764.

29. Wagner, P., Moseley, G., Grant, M., Gore, J., Owens, C. (2002) Physicians' emotional intelligence and patient satisfaction. *Family Medicine.* 34(10), 750-54.

30. Stein, S., Book, H. (2011) *The EQ edge: Emotional intelligence and your success.* 3rd ed. Mississauga, Ont. Jossey-Bass.

31. Eisenberger NI. Why rejection hurts: what social neuroscience has revealed about the brain's response to social rejection. In: Decety J, Cacioppo J, editors. *The Handbook of Social Neuroscience.* New York, NY: Oxford. University Press; 2011:109Y27.

32. Moreno-Jiménez B., Barbaranelli C., Herrer MG., Hernández EG. (2012) The physician burnout questionnaire: A new definition and measure. *TPM - Testing, Psychometrics, Methodology in Applied Psychology, 19*(4), 325-344. DOI: 10.4473/TPM19.4.6.

33. Gardner H. (1983) *Frames of Mind.* Basic Books. Underlining and Notation edition (1983).

34. EQi 2.0 User's Handbook 2011, Toronto Canada: Multi Health System.

35. Salovey P., Mayer J. D. (1990). Emotional intelligence. *Imagination, Cognition, and Personality.* 9, 185-211. doi:0.2190/DUGG-P24E-52WK-6CDG.

36. Goleman D. (1995) *Emotional intelligence: Why it can matter more than IQ.* Bloomsbury; 12.2.1995 edition.

37. Goleman D. (2000) *Working with Emotional Intelligence.* Bantam; Reprint edition.

38. https://www.kornferry.com/institute/647-a-better-return-on-self-awareness

39. https://atrium.haygroup.com/downloads/marketingps/nz/ESCI_research_findings_2010.pdf

40. Codier E, Kooker BM, Shoultz J. (2008) Measuring the emotional intelligence of clinical staff nurses: an approach for improving the clinical care environment. *Nursing Administration.* 32(1), 8-14.

41. Morrison J. (2008) The relationship between emotional intelligence competencies and preferred conflict-handling styles. *Journal of Nursing Management.* 16(8), 974-83.

42. Zhu Y., Liu C., Guo B., Zhao L., Lou F. (2015) The impact of emotional intelligence on work engagement of registered nurses: the mediating role of organisational justice. *Journal of Clinical Nursing.* 24(15-16):2115-24.

43. Mandel, E.D., Schweinle, W.E. (2012) A study of empathy decline in physician assistant students at completion of first didactic year. *The Journal of Physician Assistant Education.* 23(4), 16-24.

44. Freshman B., Rubino L. (2002) Emotional Intelligence: A Core Competency for Health Care Administrators. *Health Care Manager.* 20(4), 1–9.

45. Balch C.M., Freischlag J.A., Shanafelt T.D. (2009) Stress and burnout among surgeons: understanding and managing the syndrome and avoiding the adverse consequences. *Archives of Surgery.* 144(4):371-6. doi: 10.1001/archsurg.2008.575.

46. Orsekovich M., Anderson J. (2013) Physician personalities and burnout. *Bulletin of the American College of Surgeons.* 98(6):40-2.

47. Gordon C.E., Borkan S.C. (2014) Recapturing time: a practical approach to time management for physicians. *Postgraduate Medical Journal.* 90(1063), 267-72.

48. Epstein RM, Krasner MS. (2013) *Physician Resilience: what it means, why it matters, and how to promote it.* Academic Medicine. 88(3), 301-3.

49. Quoidbach, Mikolajczak and Gross (2015) Positive Interventions: An Emotion Regulation Review. *Psychological Bulletin*, American Psychological Association.

50. Cialdini, R. (2016) *Pre-Suasion: A Revolutionary Way to Influence and Persuade.* New York: Simon and Shuster.

51. https://www.kornferry.com/institute/filling-your-blind-spots

52. Davidson and Begley (2012): *Emotional Life of Your Brain.* New York: Penguin Group.

53. Newberg A. and Waldman, M.R. (2012). *Words Can Change Your Brain.* New York: Penguin Group.

54. Covey S. (2013) *The 7 Habits of Highly Effective People: Powerful lessons in personal change.* Simon & Schuster; Anniversary edition.

55. McGonical K. (2015) *The upside of stress, why stress is good for you, and how to get good at it.* Penguin Random House: New York.

56. http://www.wellcoach.com/memberships/images/Chapter-12.pdf

ABOUT THE AUTHOR

• • •

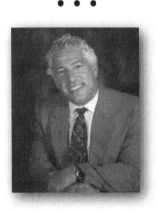

CLINICAL PSYCHOLOGIST AND EXECUTIVE COACH, Reldan Nadler, PsyD, MCC, has over thirty years' experience coaching high-performing executives and their teams. The author of several best-selling books on leadership, Dr. Nadler provides services to physicians' groups regarding the implementation of emotional-intelligence techniques. He has developed and pioneered EI-based programs for physicians and healthcare professionals.

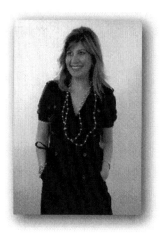

Zeina Ghossoub El-Aswad, PhD, CPEC, PCC, CWC, holds a master's degree in human nutrition and a doctorate in human behavior. A best-selling author, she has ten years' experience as a wellness coach and executive coach and regularly works with major physician groups. A national and international figure, she has developed and implemented wellness and self-care programs that target physicians and healthcare professionals.

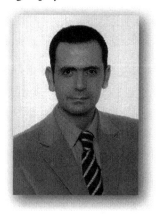

Naim El-Aswad, MD, is a pioneer in the realm of physician burnout. He has researched, presented, advised, consulted, published, and developed programs on burnout. He has practiced internal and emergency medicine for over seventeen years.

The authors provide a timely, comprehensive analysis of physician burn out – a topic everybody involved in healthcare must be very familiar with. More, they make a compelling case to get out of this crisis. A highly recommended read for any physician.

Armin A. Zadeh MD PhD MPH Johns Hopkins University

I like the easily digestible chapters and overall flow of the book. For busy practitioners especially, it provides high yield information with credible resources as a sort of practical "tool kit"...I think "cancer" analogy is very relatable.

Lara Colton, MD, FACP
Associate Residency Program Director
Assistant Professor of Internal Medicine
Weill Cornell Medical College

"This book is a call to action for our profession, indeed, an entire industry! Dr. El-Aswad et al employ the metaphor of malignancy to illuminate the prevalence, dangers, and clinical presentation of healthcare provider burnout. The metaphor extends to the provocative suggestion that we screen providers for burnout starting as early as medical school and continuing throughout our careers as well as proposals for a rigorous treatment plan. Cogent, well-researched, and thought-provoking, it is a valuable read for anyone concerned about provider health and sustainability."

Fabienne Moore, MD MPH

Made in the USA
San Bernardino, CA
08 April 2018